PRAISE FOR
UNDUE BURDEN
& DR. TAYLOR

"Dr. DeShawn Taylor is a true physician activist, and this book is a clarion call for action. Dr. Taylor's unique perspective as a physician who provides abortions *and* engages with her community informs every chapter. This timely book outlines her vision for a more just society and how activism around abortion access, at every level, moves us closer to that vision, in spite of the overturning of *Roe v. Wade.*

"Avoiding the usual and problematic polarized rhetoric around abortion, Dr. Taylor outlines how we have to move from a mindset of 'I'm pro-choice, but …' to 'I embrace a future in which all people have access to the healthcare that they need.'"

—SUSAN YANOW
Cofounder, Women Help Women

"Dr. DeShawn Taylor has written an important book. It will be a balm to so many who are trying to understand the debate about abortion and gain clarity about their own views. From her perspective as a physician, a Black woman, and a person of faith, she brings elements that many previous books on the topic have not included but that people I have spoken with over my decades-long involvement with reproductive self-determination sincerely want to know. It is well past time to stop defending abortion rights as an issue separate from the whole person and a woman's right to define her place in the world. Dr. Taylor's proposal for a new narrative could not be more urgently needed."

—GLORIA FELDT
Cofounder and president, Take the Lead

"Dr. Taylor has written nothing short of an abortion-care manifesto by providing an entirely new prism from which to address the attack on abortion rights in America. She challenges those in the traditional reproductive rights space to think bigger by arguing that, even while intact, *Roe* was never enough. In so doing she uncovers the true limitations of 'choice' while also uncovering why the current post-*Roe* response remains woefully inadequate as it, in practice, still leaves millions behind. Instead, she offers a bold new vision to move us beyond a narrow focus on reproductive rights in favor of a much more expansive vision of creating a new reality in America, which is truly reflective of reproductive justice. Perhaps her call will spur the type of movement that's necessary to finally produce true reproductive freedom in America, once and for all."

—AVIS JONES-DEWEEVER, PHD
Senior policy advisor, Black Women's Roundtable

"Dr. Taylor's training, expertise, and deep compassion for the patients she cares for is apparent in each word she writes. Her analysis is as complicated as the lives of her patients. As we grapple with the future before us, one where our bodily agency and autonomy are under constant threat, Dr. Taylor has shared with us a road map for the way forward, and it is reproductive justice!"

–JAMILA PERRITT, MD, MPH, FACOG
President and CEO, Physicians for Reproductive Health

"Dr. DeShawn Taylor was divinely inspired to start her own medical practice and equally inspired to write this book. Just as it has been her desire that anyone who comes into her clinic would be blessed, anyone who reads *Undue Burden* will be blessed. She provides a holistic and integrative approach to reproductive healthcare and calls physicians, faith leaders, and all of us to the important action of bringing integrated reproductive justice approaches to our service in the world. *Undue Burden* gives readers the theological, sociological, and medical frameworks to challenge the conservative Christian narratives that have oppressed bodily autonomy, disrupted spiritual agency, and damned people to hell in the process. We should all be grateful that Dr. Taylor is no longer silent about being a provider of faith."

–REV. DR. CARI JACKSON
Religious Coalition for Reproductive Choice

"I feel like I've just taken a shot of reality versus my perception. I never realized how the narrative was framed around the word *pro-choice*, but if I am honest, it makes perfect sense. The way Dr. Taylor concludes each chapter with myths and reality shone a light into my own belief systems and is causing me to take a deep look at myself and the conversation I deploy when operating as an advocate for change in this space. I am grateful to have the opportunity to self-reflect on what I truly believe in contrast to what I've simply adopted as truth with no merit."

—ALYCIA HUSTON
Founder and CEO, The Culture Cru

UNDUE BURDEN

UNDUE BURDEN

A **Black, Woman** Physician
on Being **Christian**
and **Pro-Abortion** in the
Reproductive Justice Movement

DESHAWN TAYLOR, MD

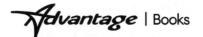 | Books

Published by Advantage, Charleston, South Carolina.
Member of Advantage Media.

ADVANTAGE is a registered trademark, and the Advantage colophon is a trademark of Advantage Media Group, Inc.

Printed in the United States of America.

10 9 8 7 6 5 4 3 2 1

ISBN: 978-1-64225-659-8 (Paperback)
ISBN: 978-1-64225-658-1 (eBook)

LCCN: 9781642256598

Cover design by Matthew Morse.
Layout design by Matthew Morse.

This publication is designed to provide accurate and authoritative information in regard to the subject matter covered. It is sold with the understanding that the publisher is not engaged in rendering legal, accounting, or other professional services. If legal advice or other expert assistance is required, the services of a competent professional person should be sought.

Advantage Media helps busy entrepreneurs, CEOs, and leaders write and publish a book to grow their business and become the authority in their field. Advantage authors comprise an exclusive community of industry professionals, idea-makers, and thought leaders. Do you have a book idea or manuscript for consideration? We would love to hear from you at **AdvantageMedia.com**.

For my father, who I wish were here to read these pages.
This daddy's girl grew up to be the confident and fearless woman I am
because of my father's love.

For my mother, one of the most courageous women I know.
We've grown to know each other more intimately during these
twenty-one years that I have been an abortion provider.

CONTENTS

ACKNOWLEDGMENTS

I would like to acknowledge my small but mighty clinical team: Karlee, Rose, and Rui, who have continued to come to work against some of the greatest odds. Thank you for trusting my vision and remaining dedicated to delivering just, dignified, and exceptional care.

Volunteers helped us show up consistently to serve. Brian, Harlie, Jo, Melody, R., and Rachel, my heart overflows with gratitude for you. Brian and Melody, we would literally not be able to provide surgical abortion services without you.

Najima, you are such a fierce supporter from afar, coordinating the very first fundraiser supporting the operations of the Desert Star clinic. Willbliss commissioned a sketch of me on a canvas that the community painted and presented to me at the close of the event. My heart was and continues to be full then and now when I think about that day.

The doors of the clinic remain open with financial support from community donations and grants from the Abortion Care Network's Keep Our Clinics fund. Nancy, your donation allowed me to make payroll and pay the lease. I did a happy dance when I opened up the envelope with your check in it. I remain in awe of your generosity.

To everyone who prayed, offered encouraging words, helped out on a project here or there, referred someone for care, defended my honor against the haters on social media, and all other acts of love, knowing and unknowing, thank you for holding me down.

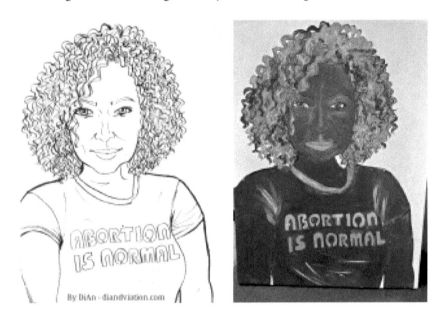

Left: The commissioned sketch by DiAn (diandviation.com).
Right: The finished canvas painted by the community at the Desert Star fundraiser.

FOREWORD

"You have to center reproductive justice … working with clinics like Desert Star … and physicians like Dr. DeShawn Taylor."

Abolitionist and activist Alejandra Pablos is speaking to a room of over five hundred reproductive health professionals. This is not the first time I have heard Dr. Taylor's name mentioned in the large conferences and meetings of worried and determined reproductive health, rights, and justice professionals after the fall of *Roe*.

Abortion Care Network is the only national US-based membership organization devoted to the needs and visibility of independent abortion providers. My role is to support these abortion clinics in providing the majority of abortion care in the United States. I sit in the back of this conference room to continue scribbling my notes on the next steps in the intersectional fight for reproductive justice in this "new" landscape, specifically about criminalization. I feel relieved to know that Dr. DeShawn Taylor's name was mentioned. Because I know she has thought through and been through some of the most challenging aspects of abortion care in our country. She knows the insanity of the moving target of abortion provision, understands the nuance of healthcare versus the black-or-white narrative of choice, and is deeply committed to humanity and uncovering the histories of reproductive coercion, misinformation, genocide, and violence of an emboldened antiabortion movement.

Although the only Black physician owner of an abortion clinic in the red state of Arizona, I don't hear Dr. DeShawn Taylor's name, voice, or perspective often enough. But both Alejandra and DeShawn are in Arizona. While they both have two very different stories, this is a shared mission of liberation. Over the years, I have sat with Dr. Taylor as she continued to meet the barriers and challenges that were distinctly due to her identity and the assumptions about who she was. The reproductive justice movement is a home for many; however, physicians face many obstacles, and with constant legal battles, they tend to be isolated—much like abortion. Patients and providers are asked to face insurmountable barriers and burdens, and the overpoliticization, constant interference, and cultural rhetoric are a targeted binary that is unrealistic and unsustainable as we live our whole lives.

Alejandra continues speaking to the room of at least five hundred, emphasizing her intersectionality as an abortion patient, a detainee of ICE, and a multilingual activist at the borders of the US. Dr. Taylor is not in the room, and I know exactly where she is—providing abortion care to her community.

In 2020 Dr. Taylor won the Maricopa County NAACP Trailblazer Award for "outstanding Leadership in the Health Field and tremendous community service." She spoke of the power of reproductive justice. I talk to Dr. Taylor at least once a month, hearing her ever-present spirit and the voice of someone who can, someone who will, and someone who walks on a pathway forward that is full of abundance and community. Every interaction and conversation are about care, patient care, expanding care, caring for her staff, or building community. Her ability to both provide and to lead is unique and is powerful.

With the fall of *Roe*, now it's time to hear from a provider, an educator, a mentor, and a physician activist living and working in a state that has lost what little access they had. Dr. Taylor beautifully shows us how to support abortion now and for generations by modeling conversations, principles, and lifelong work based on reproductive justice, boundless courage, deep learning, abundance, and curiosity instead of fear.

—ERIN GRANT
Co—executive director, Abortion Care Network

INTRODUCTION

Someone is shouting at my receptionist.

The angry voice reaches me as I come out of an exam room in the back of my gynecology and family planning clinic in Phoenix, Arizona. I am an ob-gyn (obstetrician-gynecologist) who provides abortions, so you might guess that the yelling is coming from an anti-abortion fanatic, but you'd be wrong. The voice I hear is a desperate woman, suddenly come face to face with the reality of abortion care in an American state hostile to abortion rights.

I can't believe I have to wait. I can't believe I have to pay. I can't believe my insurance doesn't cover it. Why won't you help me?

Several times a week somebody is verbally abusing my receptionist because of the hoops they have to jump through to receive abortion care in our state. And hey, I get it. I'm angry too. I often have to bring my staff together for a pep talk to deal with this reality. We remind one another that folks are just out there living their lives. They're not thinking about the fact that one day they may become the one woman in four who will have an abortion in America before the age of forty-five. (As a quick note: Throughout this book I will use the terms *woman/women, pregnant person/people,* or *people who can become pregnant*, acknowledging that transgender and nonbinary people become pregnant, have abortions, and need access to reproductive healthcare.)

Many of the people who show up in my office don't even know what *Roe v. Wade* was. Maybe you're not entirely sure either. I get it. The "my body, my choice" conversation is not one that often touches people where they live, on the ground, so when they enter the world of reproductive healthcare—my world—they're often plenty surprised and angry at what they find.

Honestly, the world of abortion care is moving so swiftly, even I struggle to keep up. As I sat down to write this introduction in May of 2022, a leaked draft of the *Dobbs v. Jackson Women's Health Organization* Supreme Court decision told those of us who were listening that *Roe v. Wade* would likely be struck down.[1] I'd like to pause to mark that extraordinary moment. We were given a warning, a glimpse into a future when 33.6 million American people who can become pregnant would lose access to legal abortion care.[2] Three months later, *Dobbs* became law, and *Roe* was gone. The US Constitution was held to no longer protect a person's right to abortion. Three months after that, as I penned my conclusion to this book, my home state of Arizona revived an 1864 law from before Arizona was even a state that made providing abortion care illegal except to save the life of the pregnant person. By the time you read these words, the law likely will have changed again.

I will not break the law. I did not go to medical school to go to jail. I have no interest in performing illegal abortions, ever. As

---

1   Josh Gerstein and Alexander Ward, "Supreme Court Has Voted to Overturn Abortion Rights, Draft Opinion Shows," Politico, May 2, 2022, https://www.politico.com/news/2022/05/02/supreme-court-abortion-draft-opinion-00029473.

2   "American Community Survey 2016-2020 5-Year Data Release," Center for Reproductive Rights, Guttmacher Institute, March 17, 2022, https://www.census.gov/newsroom/press-kits/2021/acs-5-year.html.

a Black woman, I have no illusions about what types of risks I can take. I know that if a provider was targeted with criminal penalties for helping someone access abortion care, there's a good chance it would be me. The question I ask myself now is, How do I advocate for pregnant people who need my help when the laws change from moment to moment?

My answer to that question—in part—is this book. I started thinking about writing this book as I grappled with the likelihood that the Supreme Court would overturn *Roe v. Wade*, months before that leaked draft opinion ever surfaced. I've always been an advocate for women, and more specifically, those who are poor and marginalized. I won't stop that fight now. Our opposition has played a long game that many Americans didn't realize they were in until they were desperately playing catch-up. The courts were intentionally packed with judges who will not protect us. Politicians were intentionally groomed to take our rights away. Although a bit disillusioned at times, I have not lost hope. In the words of Dr. Martin Luther King Jr., "the arc of the moral universe is long, but it bends toward justice."

The good news is that the road map for how to move forward already exists. There is a better way, and it's working already. I've seen it in my practice, in my community, and in my life.

How We Got Here

The definition of insanity is doing the same thing over and over and expecting a different result. For the five decades after *Roe v. Wade*, we've continued to talk about abortion rights as a woman's individual right to privacy, the individual's right to have abortion care without governmental interference. "My body, my choice" is not wrong. It got us *Roe*, and that's been good. But even with *Roe*, it's estimated that eleven million women of reproductive age lived over an hour from an abortion clinic,[3] making legal abortion access impossible due to poverty and other restraints. Since I started providing abortion care in Arizona in 2009, every year but one there has been a new abortion restriction signed into law.

What good was a "right" to privacy if pregnant people still couldn't get the legal abortions they needed, especially the poor and people of color who are most hurt by these restrictions? Talking about *bodily rights* was too abstract. Siloing abortion care into its own space, separate from other rights, wasn't working. Abortion opponents have been too successful in framing the conversation. What we did before is what brought us to where we are now—this place of extreme, uneven, and unfair restrictions on care that disproportionately hurt the most vulnerable among us.

We have to open our eyes to what's happening on the ground. That means looking through a different lens. We need a new narrative and a new language to describe what we see. Luckily, we already have that in the framework of reproductive justice. Don't worry if you don't know what that means. Most people don't. A new language needs to be learned, piece by piece. This book will lay out the path.

By the time you're done reading these pages, you will understand how reproductive justice can give the over 60 percent of people who support abortion rights a new way to talk about their convictions.[4] It can give the 24 percent of people who will get an abortion before the age of forty-five in America a better way to think and to speak

---

3   K. K. Rebecca Lai and Jugal K. Patel, "For Millions of American Women, Abortion Access Is Out of Reach," *New York Times*, May 31, 2019, https://www.nytimes.com/interactive/2019/05/31/us/abortion-clinics-map.html.

4   Jeff Diamant and Besheer Mohamed, "What the Data Says about Abortion in the U.S.," June 24, 2022, Pew Research Center, https://www.pewresearch.org/fact-tank/2022/06/24/what-the-data-says-about-abortion-in-the-u-s-2/.

out about their experiences.[5] It outlines how we can move beyond being pro-choice to being proabortion, what that means, and why that matters.

This book is a call to action. In its pages, I'll explain what reproductive justice is, why it differs from the current abortion rights conversation, and how you can actively get involved. Along the way, we'll talk about trans men and nonbinary people, the idea of Black genocide, the idea of adoption as a substitute for abortion, disability rights, the role of race, and perhaps most importantly in our current political climate, how Christian extremism has convinced society that abortion is the ultimate sin, despite what those of us who are spiritual truly know about God. Also, I will give you a behind the scenes view of what it looks like on the front lines of caring for people who can become pregnant and fighting for reproductive justice from the point of view of a Black cis woman, practicing Christian, and ob-gyn medical doctor who owns her own family planning clinic.

My vision for this book is realized when those who need reproductive care, those who love and care for them, and those who provide care come together to acknowledge that our oppressions are interconnected. Only then can we center the real-life experiences of people impacted by harmful policies and work together to create better lives, healthier families, and sustainable communities.

—DR. DESHAWN TAYLOR

---

5   "Abortion Is a Common Experience for U.S. Women, Despite Dramatic Declines in Rates," Guttmacher Institute, Oct 19, 2017, https://www.guttmacher.org/news-release/2017/abortion-common-experience-us-women-despite-dramatic-declines-rates.

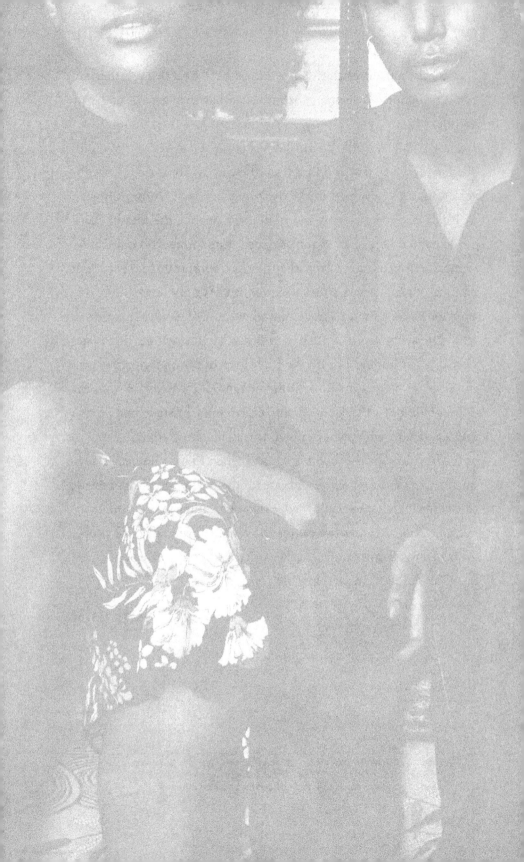

CHAPTER ONE

RECONCILING HEART AND MIND

The Rhetoric of Pro-Life and Pro-Choice, and How to Fight It

Cheryl, a partnered woman in her thirties, came into our clinic for abortion care.[6] She completed her initial consultation for an abortion without incident. At my clinic this includes the patient completing a worksheet that we talk through with them to explore their thoughts and feelings about receiving abortion care, an ultrasound to confirm and date the pregnancy, a routine review of their chosen abortion procedures and what to expect, and state-mandated, scripted information that has to be provided to the patient in person by a physician. Because Arizona requires people to wait twenty-four hours after the initial consultation, she returned a different morning for her chosen surgical abortion procedure. Again, she seemed still resolute in her

---

6   Throughout this book, names and minor identifying details are changed to protect privacy.

decision. That's typical, because when minds are made up, waiting rarely changes things.

She received medications to induce what we call a "twilight state" of semiconsciousness to ease any discomfort, similar to what you might experience in the dentist's office for a root canal. As we prepared to begin, she grew agitated and upset. This sometimes happens as people experience a loss of control as the sedatives start to take effect, but I pay close attention. When people are conscious, they can create the mental conditions that allow them to go through with something that they've convinced themselves that they need to do. I believe sedation strips away the ability to do that and exposes what lies just beneath their conscious thought. I couldn't be sure what was going on with Cheryl. Sometimes, things can bubble up under sedation that have nothing to do with the procedure. For example, if someone has experienced previous trauma, that can surface under the sedative drugs. But other times, what I'm seeing is repressed emotional distress about the abortion itself. Either way, I needed Cheryl to be sure she was okay before we moved forward—and I needed to be sure too. So I stopped what I was doing and let Cheryl know that I had not done anything to disrupt the pregnancy and asked her if she wanted me to proceed. She said, "No."

We stopped the procedure and took Cheryl to the recovery room. She was a bit embarrassed and apologized multiple times. She felt as if she had wasted our time. I told her, "No, no. You don't have to apologize. From your behavior while sedated, I was concerned that today maybe wasn't the day for you to have an abortion."

She ultimately shared, "I really want to have this abortion, but emotionally, I'm just not ready."

Emotionally, I'm just not ready.

I don't want to talk anyone into or out of an abortion.
I only want them to be aware of how they feel and why.

The majority of people coming into our clinic are fine with their choice, both in heart and mind. In fact, every day, people come to my clinic who are pretty happy about the fact that they're about to have their abortion because their life was on a path, and they want to stay on that path. Others, like Cheryl, have also rationally decided that bringing another child into the world at this time in their life is not the right thing to do, and yet, they still feel emotionally conflicted in ways that they're often not aware of and that they can't express in words. People need to put language to how they're feeling, especially if they're having a difficult time making a decision.

In this chapter, I'll explore the most common conflicts that I've seen people experience around their decisions to have abortions. I will argue that these conflicts are often caused by external, societal narratives that people have deeply internalized but that they haven't thought much about and often do not truly believe once they do. Uncovering and interrogating these narratives helps people find the language to untangle what's going on inside them.

I want people making the decision to have an abortion
to be at peace with their choice.

I consider my medical practice to be my ministry. As a deeply spiritual person, I feel called to attend to all aspects of my patients' well-being when they're in my care. That morning Cheryl left the clinic. She returned a couple of weeks later, and a surgical abortion was completed. The high level of anxiety that Cheryl exhibited previously was gone. She had taken additional time to reconcile her heart and mind and, in doing so, found her own personal truth.

I hope after reading this chapter, you'll be able to identify where your own personal mind-heart conflicts lie around the issue of abortion and to do the same.

"Am I Going to Hell?"

Narrative: Getting an abortion is a sin against God.

The rhetoric of the antiabortion movement is powerful, especially for people who have faith. People who are personally religiously conflicted and considering abortion are often trying to reconcile the fact that they're considering an abortion with what they understand about their faith—that they're not supposed to be doing this. There's a wide spectrum of belief, but the most in-distress people ask me directly, "Am I going to hell?"

As a practicing Christian who believes in God, I have a lot to say on the topic. In chapter 2, I'll go deeper into the distorted religious narratives created around abortion and why they exist. But for now, and in the exam room, I keep it simple and direct. (Because most of my patients are Christian, that's what I'll address in this chapter. Chapter 2 addresses the beliefs of other faiths.)

When someone is particularly religious, I discuss how there is no specific passage in the Bible that says abortion is bad. A lot of Christians will bring up Jeremiah 1:5: "Before I formed you in the womb, I knew you." I tell them that Christianity preaches that the body is just a vessel. I say, "Know that if God wants a spirit to get to Earth, then he's going to put it in somebody else. You can remove yourself. You can take that burden away from yourself."

When the issue of "life begins at conception" arises, a topic we'll discuss the biology and history of in chapter 2, I say, "The Bible says that God brings life into us when we're born. Genesis 2:7 reads: He 'breathed into his nostrils the breath of life and it was then that the man became a living being.'" I tell them that they are carrying a potential life and so their actual wants, needs, and desires trump those of the potential life that's growing inside them. I say, "You get to create the life that you have a vision of. You don't have to throw it away because you've become unintentionally pregnant."

The idea of abortion as the ultimate sin is also common. To this I say, "If someone commits a sin, then they're supposed to repent, to ask God for forgiveness, and then they're forgiven. Do you not believe that applies to you? Someone can commit actual murder of a living human being, and we believe that that person can be redeemed. They can repent and ask for forgiveness from God. So why is it that you deciding to have an abortion is any different? I don't believe that what's happening here is a sin, but if you do, then why don't you believe that you can ask God for forgiveness, repent, and be forgiven? Only He knows your heart."

Some people, however, are so deeply committed to the narrative of religious persecution and to their persecuted state they can't be reached. It sometimes seems as though people come into the clinic trying to create scenarios where their persecution is validated. I ponder what they may be thinking: *I'm hating myself right now because I'm considering having an abortion. I want you to treat me poorly, so then I can continue to be mad at myself and you too.* I remind staff, and myself, that we can't take it personally. The way people are behaving has nothing to do with us. And we never want to escalate the situation.

When people show up this way, I say, "I don't believe you're committing sin. I sleep fine at night providing abortion care, and I believe in God. But if you believe you're committing a sin, then don't do it." They say, "Oh, but I have to do it." So then I say, "Well, no, you don't. If we can't come up with any moral argument that makes you feel better about this, then don't do it." Some people will leave and take some time. Other people will say, "You know what, I'm gonna have my abortion."

To me, this shows that at the center of it all, most people innately know that they have ultimate say over their bodies and their lives. They're here in my clinic, after all, exercising their autonomy to make this decision that they believe in despite the narratives that barrage them from outside themselves. They understand that they have the instinctive, inborn ability to control their fertility as people with uteruses have for thousands of years and as they will continue to do for thousands of years to come, no matter the barriers thrown in their path. They understand on some level that being human means controlling the trajectory of their lives, and for this one moment, they gather the strength to put away the opinions of others and listen to their heart.

MOST PEOPLE INNATELY KNOW THAT THEY HAVE ULTIMATE SAY OVER THEIR BODIES AND THEIR LIVES.

In later chapters, we'll look more deeply at the reasons people's lived, true experiences often conflict with what they're told on certain topics, including racism, sexism, misogyny, paternalism, economic discrimination, and so on. For now, just know that listening to your heart is hard, we all do the best we can, and just being aware of the narratives that don't ring true in our souls is a good place to start.

The Problem of Other People

Narrative: Abortion is rare, the exception;
only "bad" people get them.

For many religious and nonreligious people, their distress often does not come from imagined persecution from God but from other people who claim to be moral authorities. They say, "I don't want people to judge me." I assure them that they probably already know and love someone who's had an abortion, because abortion is very common. People just don't talk about it. I urge them to consider that they will probably be surprised at the support they might receive if they do decide to share their decision to have an abortion with the people they love.

> One in four women will have an abortion in their reproductive lifetime.[7] Over 60 percent of these are people of faith.[8]

The dominant, public narrative that abortions are rare and shameful is not the truth of people's lives. Often, the people I see in the worst emotional shape are the people who have been loudly and aggressively antiabortion but are now in my clinic to get their own abortions. I often have to console distressed and crying people who are now reckoning with how poorly they treated someone else whom they care about. One tearful woman shared, "I was so horrible to my sister when she did this, and now here I am. I am such a horrible person. I cannot believe I'm here." I always tell people, "You never know what

---

7   Guttmacher Institute, "Abortion Is a Common Experience."

8   Rachel K. Jones, "People of All Religions Use Birth Control and Have Abortions," Guttmacher Institute, October 2020, https://www.guttmacher.org/article/2020/10/people-all-religions-use-birth-control-and-have-abortions?gclid=CjwKCAjwp9qZBhBkEiwAsYFsb15G0e7cLh5WeaiCekh Bu8rSvxtzBKjloDDFthLU4FtdayUDAZiU3xoCkV8QAvD_BwE.

you would do until you're faced with the choice." Ultimately, I hope that they can go back to the people they have hurt and reconcile. I tell them, "I'm not here to judge you or treat you poorly because you did that to somebody else. I'm here to take care of you."

The Problematic Rhetoric of Pro-Choice
Narrative: There are good and bad abortions.

Many people don't realize how problematic and harmful the rhetoric of the pro-choice movement can be both to themselves and to others who will one day need abortion care.

I use birth control. I don't sleep around. I was very careful. We use condoms all the time. I can't believe I'm here. I wouldn't be here except ...

This is often what I hear from people who tell me they're pro-choice, and it's the qualifications that cause problems. Katha Pollitt, in her book *Pro,* calls these people the "muddled middle."[9] These are the "millions of Americans—more than half—who don't want to ban abortion exactly, but don't want it to be widely available either." It's an attitude of "permit but discourage." They accept the narrative that there is "grief, shame, and stigma" in ending their pregnancies, while also claiming that it's just fine for others. In other words, Pollitt explains, they believe "you can have your abortion as long as you feel really, really bad about it."[10] In fact, pro-choice people in my office for their abortions sometimes ask me, "How do you do this?" Even though they claim to be openminded and pro-choice, they want me to feel as bad about abortion as they do.

I will not. For these people, just as for the so-called pro-life folks, I want to help them reconfigure the narrative. I believe that abortion

---

9   Katha Pollitt, Pro (New York: Picador, 2014), 36.

10   Pollitt, Pro, 37.

is a positive, moral choice. All people who can become pregnant want to thrive, not just survive. They want opportunity. They want to finish school. They want to keep that job that they're about to lose because their pregnancy is making them so sick they can no longer go to work. They want to provide for the children they already have.

> When we say abortion saves lives, it literally saves lives. But it also saves lives in the sense of saving the life that someone has that will be completely derailed should they not get their abortion.

Many pro-choice advocates often don't believe that abortion is a positive social good in this way, even though they say they support access to abortion care. I want people to get beyond the pro-choice narrative and become proabortion. Whether they would choose to have an abortion themselves is not relevant to the discussion.

I also want people to be aware of how the pro-choice discussion reinforces the narrative of good vs. bad abortions. As Bill Clinton expressed it, he wanted to make abortion "safe, legal, but rare."[11] But why rare? That only stigmatizes what is a common procedure and gives abortion opponents the opportunity to regulate abortion care out of existence. Abortion doesn't have to be a tragedy. If a person wants to have an abortion for whatever reason, they should have an abortion, without shame or having to justify themselves. The pro-choice narrative casts a dark shadow of shame, guilt, and qualification that muddles the idea of choice.

In my clinic, I tell my pro-choice patients, "Extend yourself some grace. You're human. Mistakes happen. Honestly you have about

---

11   Bill Clinton, Executive Orders Signing, Abortion Rights and Medical Research Orders, January 22, 1993, C-Span, https://www.c-span.org/video/?37335-1/abortion-rights-medical-research-orders.

thirty years of your life when you can become pregnant, and you seem to have done a pretty good job not being pregnant until now. All we can do is make our best effort, and there is nothing that will completely prevent pregnancy besides not having sex. And wouldn't that be such a boring life?"

I hope through these words, the pro-choice people in my care will extend that grace to others and so will you.

A New Narrative

Identifying and processing harmful, untrue narratives around abortion helps people reconcile their hearts and minds. But this is just the first step. The important work that comes next is to replace these old narratives with a new framework for thinking about abortion. The emotional distress that arises when our realities don't mesh with the stories we're being told can only be truly healed when we uncover a new narrative that does.

In the next chapters, we'll explore more deeply some religious narratives around abortion and their intersections with racism, sexism, white supremacy, and patriarchy. In exploring these issues, you will begin to understand how reproductive justice is a framework that gives us a different way to think about how we decide if, when, and how to have children and raise families. It takes the conversation from pro-choice to proabortion, from blame to a celebration of possibility, and from individual responsibility to the responsibilities of the community.

It's a challenge to reconfigure your thinking. But the work of doing so doesn't only help your own situation; it can be the beginning of healing our very broken and divisive world.

TALKING THROUGH NARRATIVES

Myth: Choosing abortion is a purely rational decision.

Reality: "Talking through why I felt so much shame about my abortion made me realize I was actually doing the right thing for me."

Myth: Abortion is an unforgivable sin.

Reality: "I believe in God. I go to church, I pray. I can shut out all the noise and all the people who are telling me what to do, and I can have a personal conversation with God. I can work through this with Him because that's ultimately what matters. God knows my heart."

Myth: Abortion is always a tragedy.

Reality: "I'm already a mother, and I need to focus on the children I have. That is a positive moral choice, and so my abortion is also a positive moral choice for which I mostly feel relief."

Myth: Abortion is murder.

Reality: "The ideas of when human life begins have changed through history, even according to the church. I'll spend some time looking up the facts and decide for myself what I believe about when life begins."

Myth: Being pro-choice means I'm a good feminist.

Reality: "When I examined my mindset that abortions are okay for other people but not for me, I realized that I was setting myself apart. From now on, I'm going to pay more attention to the struggles of others and stand with them."

CHAPTER TWO

FAITH AND ABORTION CARE

My Christian faith is an identity that I have reconciled over time with the hate I have experienced at the hands of evangelical Christian extremists. Now, I amplify my faith in my work as an abortion provider.

I was raised Christian, but I wasn't raised in the dogma of Christianity. My family was spiritual. We went to church occasionally. My mom has a lot of ministers and pastors in her family. We went to Bible study. We read the Bible. But we weren't fundamentalists. As a young person, I was never exposed to what a lot of evangelical children are exposed to. For example, the idea that abortion is bad wasn't a part of my reality. I never heard, *Don't ever do it. It's a sin.* Honestly, abortion was never a topic of discussion.

When I got to my residency program as an intern, I thought, *I'm an obstetrician-gynecologist, so I should take care of people who want to be pregnant and people who don't.* Of course, I was going to provide abortion care. It didn't even occur to me that I would not. After completing my first abortion procedure and discussing it with the colleagues in training with me I realized, *Wow, there are people who don't want to do abortions. They say it is because of their religion.* For some, religious beliefs were really influencing their decisions to opt out. For others, it felt like an excuse. Over the course of my career, I have learned that many people, including physicians, don't want to be subjected to the harassment that happens at the hands of fanatical Christians. And yes, it is only these extremist Christians out there actively protesting against abortion. Other religions and more mainstream Christians really aren't.

Once I became an abortion provider, the situation really upset me. I wasn't questioning whether I believed in God or not—I did. I wasn't even questioning my Christian faith. I concentrated on providing abortion care because it was in alignment with my values and my ideas about social justice. Still, I didn't want to think too much about it, because the shouting voices were just too much.

For a while, that was where I hung my hat. I put my spirituality on the back burner. I had come to Arizona from California to become the statewide medical director for a reproductive health organization. I did that for three and a half years, and then I had a short stint with another independent abortion provider in the state. A few challenges happened along the way that

I BECAME STRONGER IN MY FAITH WHEN I STARTED TO HAVE CHALLENGES IN MY LIFE.

started to put me in a place where I began to ponder my next steps.

Like most people who are spiritual, I became stronger in my faith when I started to have challenges in my life. I prayed more. I read the Bible. I started to feel really strongly about finding a church home. For me, this was all part of the many things that happen when you're growing up. I was adulting. I had to figure things out for myself. I was in transition. That's when I really started to reach back into praying, seeking God's guidance for the next step of my life. For years, people had been encouraging me to start my own practice. I really didn't want the headache, and I still don't advise it. But I knew I couldn't stay where I was.

Starting my own medical practice was divinely inspired. What I mean by that is that when I have really heavy questions on my mind, the answers come to me through meditation and prayer. Some people say they hear God. For me, it's my own voice, my own thoughts. I bring myself to a place where I've cut off external things. I'm going deep within myself to access the spirit inside myself. I think people who are deeply spiritual understand that.

When I finally understood my inner voice and said yes to my calling, the universe opened up and moved everything along for me. I decided that I was going to start Desert Star Family Planning at the end of April 2013. I incorporated the business the first week of May, and I opened the doors in September. That's how quickly it happened, and it was unheard of. I was hiring people and buying equipment before I even had the business loan. I just knew that this was going to happen. I was already signing the lease for my first location when the loan finally came from the bank. I had supplies piled up in my office manager's garage and in my mama's garage. I was ready to go.

As I leaned into it, I understood more and more why my project truly was divinely inspired. One day, my nurse was about to sedate a woman for a surgical abortion when the patient asked me if I believed in God. I told her I did, and she asked if I would say a prayer for her. I didn't even think about it. I said a prayer for her. The patient closed her eyes, a look of peace came over her face, and we did the procedure. Afterward, I asked the nurse if that had made her feel uncomfortable. She said no and added that actually the patient hadn't required much sedation.

That was the first time prayer happened, but it wasn't the last. I never asked anyone if they wanted to pray. But if patients brought it up, I would pray with them. From that point on, patients would spontaneously pray, or we would pray together. I became more comfortable with that happening.

I thought back on all those years that I had been trying to take spirituality out of my medical practice. I hadn't wanted to deal with it because I was getting messages from the antiabortion industry that when you came in here, you were leaving your spirituality behind. They were a well-funded propaganda machine that told me I was evil, although I know that I am a child of God. Their thinking had gotten to me because I had been silent about my Christian faith. Now, I began to realize that I had been silent for too long. I could walk in the light by saying *I am a provider of faith*. I didn't have to let them take that from me.

Around this time, I was illegally taped in a heavily edited video that misrepresented a story about Planned Parenthood selling fetal tissue for profit. I was one of several people videotaped. By lying about who they were, they tried to get us to say things that they could take out of context and manipulate through heavy editing to make it seem as if we were doing terrible things to fetuses during abortions and making money off it. There was a lot of press. I was even talked about on the *Sean Hannity Show*. I was advised to not respond.

That was when I went on offense, which I believe is the best defense. I had gone silent for far too long about what I believed. Now, I came back in full force. I thought, *I'm not going to let these antiabortion extremists control the conversation. I'm not yielding the moral high ground to people who lie and distort the way they did.* I believe in God. I know my Bible verses. I have actually read the Bible. I will not let these people take that away from me.

Ever since then, I've been outspoken about my faith. I even put Bible verses on the cover photo of my personal Facebook page.

Recently somebody left a message for me on Facebook, expressing that they felt I didn't get to post Bible verses since "you kill babies." I put up a post that summarized my position:

> It is very sad how extremists have hijacked the Christian faith. I pray and meditate daily. I cover myself, my staff, and my patients in prayer. I have prayed with patients in the office. There are several scriptures that keep me encouraged in my work, despite the efforts of others who attempt to shame and harass me in the name of God. One of my favorites is 2 Timothy (1:7): "For God has not given us a spirit of fear, but of power and love and of a sound mind." I am vigilant regarding my safety, but I do not fear. My heart leapt when I read the following statement in a review that a patient posted on Google: "… anyone who comes here is blessed. Desert Star Family Planning is a safe space."

I run my medical practice as my ministry. When patients want to pray, I take their hand, close my eyes, and meditate until the words come to me based on whatever is passing between me and them at that moment. It's completely individual. I work from the idea that God lives within us and that we can tap into Him to guide us. We can do that by meditating or reading the Bible or whatever someone's ritual and practice. Whether my patients believe in Christianity, Islam, Judaism—whatever their faith—I'm able to connect. We all share the belief that there is a higher power and that we are able to access that higher power as individuals and act on its message.

We can't let the Christian right hijack Christianity—or any faith—for their purposes. Extremist Christians do not have the monopoly on caring about people's spiritual needs. Fundamentalists don't have the final say on the word of God. Uncovering distortions and mistruths from those who use religion as a cloak to gain power and control takes diligence and education. The so-called pro-life movement is very good at manipulating the faithful. I have seen so much damage done in their name in my life and in my practice. Understanding their motives and tactics helps bring faith back to where it belongs—inside the heart of each person, into the work of a compassionate society, into the work of caring doctors, and out of our supposedly secular state.

The Danger of Extremist Christians

Protesters outside health clinics often hold Bibles and crosses. They shout at people that they're sinning and will go to hell. They're so loud, disruptive, and aggressive that you have to wonder how someone becomes radicalized enough to actually harass strangers when so much of what we know about Jesus preaches the opposite. I have to always be vigilant, especially in an open carry state like Arizona, because I don't know if this is the day that one of these protesters is going to act. That constant threat of harassment at the hands of a supposedly Christian person is always with me, and it's real. After my clinic opened, I thought I had gotten my first credible death threat. Only when I filed a police report did I find out that I was already in the system; while I had worked at the statewide reproductive healthcare organization, they had staff who dealt with the harassment in the background, so that I didn't even know it was happening. The National Abortion Federation reports that since 1977, there have been 11 murders, 42 bombings, 196 arsons, 491 assaults, and "thousands of incidents of criminal activities directed at patients, providers, and volunteers."[12] This is almost always done in the name of Christianity. None of it sounds very Christian to me.

As the extremist violence around clinics and doctors has grown, the antiabortion movement began to understand that it wasn't a good look for them. In addition, Christian antiabortion extremists were increasingly being tied to white nationalism—an issue we'll cover in the next chapter when we discuss race. The mainstream antiabortion movement shifted to gentler tactics to improve their image. However, despite their successful makeover on the surface, the violence continues to escalate. From just 2020 to 2021, there's been an "increase in stalking (600%), blockades (450%), hoax devices/suspicious packages (163%), invasions (129%), and assault and battery (128%)" at health clinics that provide abortion care.[13]

The irony and hypocrisy of supposedly pro-life activists being Christians and wanting to kill me is a waste of energy to try to call out. These people have joined a cult that finds purpose in raising up the mantle to protect the so-called unborn. If they really cherished life, then they would champion universal healthcare and help parents instead of trying to shame them and hurt me. They wouldn't attack Planned Parenthood, an organization that provides essential healthcare, with only 4 percent of their services nationwide related to

---

12   "National Abortion Federation Releases 2021 Violence & Disruption Report," National Abortion Federation, June 24, 2022, https://prochoice.org/national-abortion-federation-releases-2021-violence-disruption-report/.

13   "2021 Violence & Disruption Report," National Abortion Federation, June 24, 2022, 3, https://5aa1b2xfmfh2e2mk03kk8rsx-wpengine.netdna-ssl.com/wp-content/uploads/2021_NAF_VD_Stats_Final.pdf.

abortion care.[14] The idea that someone would come and attempt to take my life or the life of someone who does the work that I do because they're warriors for the so-called unborn is not Christianity as I know it. I will not give them the moral high ground, and I will not let their voices be the loudest in the room. They are in the minority, and they have ulterior motives that cannot be ignored.

What the Bible Really Says about Abortion: Not Much

It's beyond the scope of this book to argue textual interpretation. What I know is that people of all faiths have abortions. I know that their faith leaders sometimes support them and other times don't. And I know that despite what these leaders say, in the end, most people will do what they feel in their hearts.

Still, when it comes to Judaism and Christianity, the faithful look to scripture for guidance. There is nowhere in the Bible that actually mentions elective abortion. In this absence, the passages picked out by both sides to support their opposing arguments are open to many interpretations. Because of this, I urge my patients to interpret scripture through their own hearts. As we've seen throughout history, patriarchal and political interests often manipulate people of faith for their own purposes. When we look at scripture, as when we look at the rest of the debate that swirls around abortion, we need to interrogate and unpack the motives of those who want to influence us.

What are these motives? In other chapters I lay them out fully. Here, in brief: patriarchy, misogyny, and racism. Unfortunately, these elements are embedded in much religious dogma, especially Christian

---

14   Annual Report, Planned Parenthood Federation of America, 2021, PDF, 26, https://www.planned-parenthood.org/uploads/filer_public/40/8f/408fc2ad-c8c2-48da-ad87-be5cc257d370/211214-ppfa-annualreport-20-21-c3-digital.pdf.

extremism. For example: women as descendants of Eve should be punished by giving birth, they should be under the control of men, and extramarital sex is a sin. All this is perpetuated by keeping abortion illegal. Christian extremists and white nationalists share a strategic interest: preserving and enshrining white minority rule. Preserving racial hierarchies means keeping Black people poor and sick. Banning abortion achieves this. *The Turnaway Study*, landmark research by Diana Greene Foster, demonstrated that the people who were turned away from abortions compared to those who got them were less financially stable, have higher debt, were more likely to be evicted from their homes, and have children who were more often raised in poverty.[15] Many mainstream Christian groups are open minded about abortion because they believe that Jesus preached to help the poor, not make more of them.

Turning to the Bible to achieve the aims of Christian extremism will work if we don't think for ourselves. But it's not as easy as quoting Bible verses. One example of the difficulty of turning to the Bible to prove or disprove either side of the abortion debate is Exodus 21: 22–25, the only mention of harming a fetus in the Bible. I won't include the lines here, as there are many varying English translations. These lines address the issue of an accidental miscarriage caused when in the course of two men fighting one man accidentally strikes the other's pregnant wife. The husband is paid a fine if there's a miscarriage, but if the woman dies, the attacker is put to death. To most Jews, this passage seems to indicate a difference between fetal life and existent life (*nefesh*). There is extensive Jewish *Mishnah* (the written record of Jewish rabbinical law based on centuries of oral argument

---

15   Diana Greene Foster, The Turnaway Study: Ten Years, a Thousand Women, and the Consequences of Having—or Being Denied—an Abortion (New York: Scribner, 2020).

over textual interpretation) that supports this view. Also, there is some *Mishnah* that doesn't.

Jews aren't alone in debating these few lines. Early Christians interpreted this same biblical passage to mean that life began at forty days from conception. Later, the passage was used by Catholics to show that all abortion was sin. These wildly different and constantly changing interpretations are mostly based on translation differences that are much too complex and nuanced to go into here.[16] My point is this: first, there is great disagreement even within traditions; second, interpretations have shifted over time; and third, very smart people who devote their lives to these issues disagree based on their faith traditions, their culture, their grasp and facility with the language, and their motives.

Since the Bible doesn't mention abortion again, not even in the six hundred laws passed down from God to Moses, Jews and Christians as well as people of other faith traditions often look for more general religious guidance to determine the moral value of the fetus. In other words, they want to know what God says about when human life begins. That this complicated, disputed, and constantly changing religious discussion has any effect on the laws of our secular state is suspect on its face. But if you are religious, how can you decide for yourself about the issue of when life begins?

Life Begins At ...

As you might have guessed, there is no one set spiritual answer to this question.

---

16   For a full discussion of this text including an explanation of various Jewish interpretations and an excellent short history of Christian translations and their interpretations, see Rachel Biale, *Women and Jewish Law: An Exploration of Women's Issues in Halakhic Sources* (New York: Shocken Books, 1984), 219–221.

For example, according to today's Catholic church, life begins at "ensoulment," which they believe happens at conception. However, through the centuries, Catholics have believed ensoulment happened anywhere from forty days to ninety days after conception, and after three hundred years of abortion being legal in the eyes of the church, in 1869 Pope Pius IX declared it illegal from conception, a stance that has stood till this day.[17] Of course, it's estimated that one in four Americans (24 percent) who had abortions in 2014 were Catholic,[18] so what church leadership teaches and what people actually do and believe can be quite different. In fact, a 2019 Pew Research poll found that 56 percent of Catholics believed that abortion should be legal in all or most circumstances.[19] As the group Catholics for Choice puts it: "Anti-choice Catholics can be loud, but they are the minority in the church. We believe that the Catholic tradition's teachings on social justice, human dignity, and the primacy of conscience compel us to support the right to reproductive freedom."[20]

Other Christian traditions have put the moment of ensoulment at different times and for different reasons. For much of Christianity, "quickening" was long considered the beginning of life, usually around the eighteenth week and determined by the pregnant person themself. Currently, the official statement from the American Presbyterian Church holds, "We may not know exactly when human life begins." Thus, "when an individual woman faces the decision whether to terminate a pregnancy, the issue is intensely personal, and may

17   G. Hovey, "Abortion: A History," Plan Parent Rev. 5, no. 2 (Summer 1985):18–21. PMID: 12340403. https://pubmed.ncbi.nlm.nih.gov/12340403/.

18   Jones, "People of All Religions Use Birth Control and Have Abortions."

19   "U.S. Public Continues to Favor Legal Abortion, Oppose Overturning Roe v. Wade," Pew Research Center, August 29, 2019, https://www.pewresearch.org/politics/2019/08/29/u-s-public-contin-ues-to-favor-legal-abortion-oppose-overturning-roe-v-wade/.

20   "Just the Facts: Catholic Perspectives on Sex, Gender, and Reproductive Health," Catholics for Choice, PDF, 4, https://www.catholicsforchoice.org/wp-content/uploads/2022/03/CatholicsFor-ChoiceJustTheFacts.pdf.

manifest itself in ways that do not reflect public rhetoric, or do not fit neatly into medical, legal or policy guidelines. Humans are empowered by the spirit prayerfully to make significant moral choices, including the choice to continue or end a pregnancy."[21] American Baptists state, "Many American Baptists believe that, biblically, human life begins at conception, that abortion is immoral and a destruction of a human being created in God's image (Job 31:15; Psalm 139:13–16; Jeremiah 1:5; Luke 1:44; Proverbs 31:8–9; Galatians 1:15). Many others believe that while abortion is a regrettable reality, it can be a morally acceptable action and they choose to act on the biblical principles of compassion and justice (John 8:1–11; Exodus 21:22–25; Matthew 7:1–5; James 2:2–13) and freedom of will (John 16:13; Roman 14:4–5, 10–13). Many gradations of opinion between these basic positions have been expressed within our fellowship."[22]

THERE IS NO AGREEMENT EVEN WITHIN DENOMINATIONS AS TO WHEN LIFE BEGINS.

I could go on and on through each Christian denomination, but the point is clear: there is no agreement even within denominations as to when life begins.

The Jewish religion also is not in total agreement on the question of when ensoulment happens. In general, however, the Talmud (religious law based on the Torah, or Old Testament) considers a fetus part of its mother's body, and so it can be sacrificed to save the mother until "its head has come out."[23] That is, ensoulment happens at birth.

---

21   "What We Believe: Abortion/Reproductive Choice Issues," Presbyterian Church (USA), accessed September 30, 2022, https://www.presbyterianmission.org/what-we-believe/social-issues/abortion-issues/.

22   "American Baptist Resolution Concerning Abortion and Ministry in the Local Church," ReligiousInstitute.org, accessed September 30, 2022, http://religiousinstitute.org/denom_statements/american-baptist-resolution-concerning-abortion-and-ministry-in-the-local-church/.

23   Biale, *Women and Jewish Law*, 221.

In fact, it is actually required by Jewish law to sacrifice a fetus to save the mother's life up to this moment, leading to a lawsuit happening in Florida at the time of this writing against Florida's post-fifteen-week abortion ban. Rabbi Barry Silver of Congregation L'Dor Va-Dor explains that "a woman is not just entitled to have an abortion [in Judaism], she is required to have an abortion to protect her mental wellbeing, to protect her health, to protect her safety ... This law would prohibit Jewish women from practicing Jewish law."[24] Rabbi Silver told NBC News, "It's the height of chutzpah for people to tell the Jewish people what the Bible means and lecture the Jewish people on the sanctity of life ... When life begins is a fundamental religious question, and the government now is trying to answer that for everyone, based on fundamentalist Christianity."[25]

Islam has many stances on when life begins, usually placing ensoulment at 120 days. However, as Khaleel Mohammed of San Diego State University explains, "More stringent scholars rely on another tradition that states that after the first forty days, an angel endows the fetus with hearing, sight, skin, flesh and bones. This clearly indicates the formation of a human being, and to abort after this period is deemed as forbidden."[26] I once had a Muslim patient who was telling my staff that she had come in to "kill her baby." This set off alarm bells for us, as I don't perform abortions on people who are in distress or conflicted about their decision. In the end, after a bit of back and forth, she was able to explain to us that her religion was fine with what she was doing. Her English, however, wasn't strong

---

24 Jillian Kestler-D'Amours, "Religious Freedom: The Next Battleground for US Abortion Rights?" Aljazeera News, June 17, 2022, https://www.aljazeera.com/news/2022/6/17/religious-freedom-the-next-battleground-for-us-abortion-rights#main-content-area.

25 Daniel Arkin, "Rabbi Fighting Florida's Anti-Abortion Law Is on a Mission to Help Religious Groups Challenge 'Theocratic Tyranny,'" NBC News, June 28, 2022, https://www.nbcnews.com/news/us-news/rabbi-fighting-floridas-anti-abortion-law-mission-help-religious-group-rcna35812.

26 Khaleel Mohammed, "Islam and Reproductive Choice," Religious Coalition for Reproductive Choice, accessed September 30, 2022, https://rcrc.org/muslim/.

enough for her to find the right words beyond the simplest to convey her intentions.

Ensoulment in Hinduism is complicated, because Hindus believe in reincarnation, or rebirth. The soul, or jiva, doesn't correspond perfectly to our Western ideas of the soul, but in general Hindu ideas about when life begins are wrapped up in the idea that life never ends. Most Hindus allow abortion in cases of the mother's health, and the Pew Research Institute found that in 2014, 68 percent of Hindus thought abortion should be legal in all or most cases.[27]

The question of when life begins is so difficult to pinpoint because "life" as a biological process is inherently different from what theologians mean by "life." Thirty to 50 percent of fertilized eggs won't ever implant in the uterus. It is the process of implantation that establishes a pregnancy. After implantation, 15 to 20 percent of pregnancies will end naturally in miscarriage, which is known in medical terms as *spontaneous abortion.* Giving personhood to a cell or a set of cells, most of which will be destroyed in normal biological processes, feels arbitrary, even absurd. As Katha Pollitt puts it, life at conception is "an incoherent, covertly religious idea that falls apart if you look at it closely. Few people believe it, as shown by the exceptions they are willing to make."[28]

Bringing Spirituality into Abortion Care

As a person who believes in God, I want others to know that there are more providers of Christian faith like me, and I want other providers of faith to know that they're not alone. They can bring their faith into

---

27   "Views about Abortion among Hindus," Pew Research Center, accessed September 30, 2022,
       https://www.pewresearch.org/religion/religious-landscape-study/religious-tradition/hindu/
       views-about-abortion/.

28   Pollitt, Pro, 29.

encounters with patients. There is a huge, unmet need for spiritual care for people who are seeking abortions because over 60 percent of people who come to us have a faith.

> There's a huge unmet need for resources for people of faith who are seeking abortion care.

When I'm thinking about the work I do, I tell people who are confused by all the religious and pseudoscientific rhetoric floating around them, "God put a decision in you. People have free will, and therefore there's a decision before you. I am a person called to help you carry that decision out because I am fulfilling the gifts that God gave me. God would not put a decision before you that is not yours to make. There are some people who are highly religious, who as soon as they become pregnant, they know that there's a birth and parenting at the end of it. It just never crosses their mind to do otherwise. The fact that this is on your mind at all means that it is a decision that you have been allowed to make because God gave you free will."

I realize that there are a lot of providers out there who don't feel comfortable having these conversations with patients, because they're not religious or are of a different faith than their patient. I've often been asked, "How do you even know that it's something that you need to address with a patient?"

The only way to know is to actually ask. It's just a matter of a few questions on the intake form to know if there needs to be additional conversation. My question isn't "Are you religious?" My question is "What are your concerns?" If religious belief is concerning, they're often going to write "I'm concerned that people are going to judge me." Or "I don't believe in abortion because of my religion." Or "I'm pro-choice, but I never thought this was going to happen to me."

These are all signs of the need for further discussion. I will then ask them, "So tell me a little bit more about that." This is when the religion often comes out. If the provider isn't comfortable with a religious discussion, there are resources that they should have available, websites where people can go to get the support that they need if they're not able to provide that in the clinic.

The opportunity to meet someone's spiritual needs is often missed. We need to recognize that before an abortion, many people want to talk through their issues. Even when people have made up their mind logically, some people still have some soul searching and processing to come to be ready to go through the actual process of the abortion. Sometimes I tell people, "You know, maybe today's not the day." I'm not trying to be paternalistic about it, but I want them to take a few steps back when that seems to be needed.

I can understand how some providers believe this is not their business. They may think, *somebody's here for an abortion. I'm here to provide it.* Yet I can look at a person sometimes and know that proceeding with abortion care that day will probably break them. Not everyone is like this. Most people, in fact, are happy and relieved to be getting the care they need. There is nuance here. Sometimes we have to disrupt that internal talk that is going on inside of a person that colors the experience of their abortion. If I see a person is really struggling, I have to ask, "Is today the day?" Sometimes that single question is all that it takes to bring the person back to the present and the decision before them.

As an obstetrician-gynecologist, someone who's tasked with helping people through pregnancies, wanted or not, my job is to ascribe the value to the pregnancy that the pregnant person ascribes to the pregnancy. If they think it's a miracle, it's a miracle. If they think they want to terminate their pregnancy, my job is to help to the extent possible. It's not my place to ascribe my own personal values to their situation at all, period. That's not what we are supposed to do. Our offices should be safe places, judgment-free zones.

And yet, there is space for our voices when we're called on. We must do better to uncover and handle those situations. One way to do that is to recognize that our offices can be places of spiritual connection. Our gifts as physicians and as healers are to shepherd people through what for some is a difficult time in their lives. Even when people believe they're doing the right thing for themselves and their families, there is often shame and stigma because of the society we live in. As doctors, we need to see the entire person coming to us for care, accept patients where they are, and do the best we can. Although society has put abortion care into a silo, pregnant people are making holistic decisions about themselves, their families, and their lives. For some, their religion is an important part of that. When we take part in these conversations, we are taking back the moral high ground from the extremists who have pushed us out.

TALKING ABOUT RELIGION

Myth: There's no place for religion in abortion care.

Reality: "By bringing my faith and spirituality into the clinic, I can help my patients understand why Christian extremism doesn't speak for all people of faith."

Myth: There is a set moment when human life begins that all people of faith agree on.

Reality: "Faith leaders from even within the same faith disagree on when a zygote becomes a person. That their thinking is all so different and changes over time is a good indication of how complex the issue is."

Myth: Scientists all agree that life begins at conception—the moment an egg is fertilized.

Reality: "Scientists use the term life differently than religious people. A blade of grass is alive; a seed is alive; all cells are alive. Whether one single, genetically unique cell should be considered the equivalent of a human person is a matter of ethics, morals, and religion. It's a different conversation."

Myth: People of faith don't get abortions.

Reality: "Sixty percent of abortions are provided to people of faith, so I know I'm not alone in my decision."

Myth: I deserve to be judged by other people for getting an abortion.

Reality: "Only God can judge. And God forgives. If you talk to those who love you, you might be surprised by who in your circle have already made the same choice you are—after all, one in four women of reproductive age will have an abortion, and more than half of them are people of faith."

Myth: Abortion protesters speak for people of faith.

Reality: "When I discovered the links between religious extremism and white nationalism, I began to wonder just who those people were, telling me what God said."

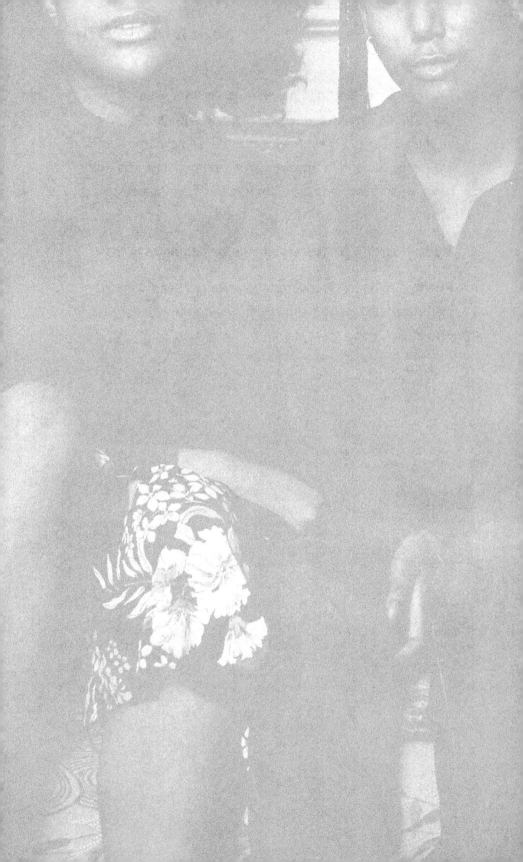

CHAPTER THREE

RACISM AND MATERNAL HEALTH

"(In) Louisiana, about a third of our population is African American. African Americans have a higher incidence of maternal mortality. So, if you correct our population for race, we're not as much of an outlier as would otherwise appear. Now, I say that not to minimize the issue, but to focus the issue as to where it would be. For whatever reason, people of color have a higher incidence of maternal mortality."

—Louisiana Senator Bill Cassidy, May 19, 2022[29]

Talk about saying the quiet part out loud. Senator Cassidy's casual dismissal of "whatever reason" one-third of his state's citizens could be dying at such alarming rates is almost as distressing as the rates themselves: American Black mothers die at three times the rate of white mothers. In Louisiana, Black mothers die at four times the rate of white mothers.

---

29   Senator Bill Cassidy, "View from the Hill: Public Health on the Brink," interview by Sarah Owermohle (Politico), Harvard Chan School of Public Health Series, accessed September 30, 2022, audio, 7:25, https://www.youtube.com/watch?v=pyqAO2CGb74/.

> Black mothers in Louisiana die at four times the rate of white mothers.[30]

Senator Cassidy's seeming bewilderment by these astonishing statistics is a dog whistle to the notion that these Black mothers who die must have done something wrong to deserve their sad fate. What we know about white supremacy and racism can fill in the blanks: they're too poor, too uneducated, probably drug users and degenerates. Their fate is their own fault due to bad genetics, poverty, and unhealthy lifestyles, and so it's not the concern of the state.

We see this attitude reflected in how the senator has dismissed other heartbreaking racial health disparities in his state. When asked why 70 percent of people who died of COVID-19 in Louisiana were Black, even though Black people made up only 32 percent of the population, the senator blamed "genetics." He said, "If you control for diabetes and hypertension, a lot of racial difference would go away. And I say that not to dismiss the problem of health disparities. We have to focus on health disparities, but we can't get distracted by that."[31]

Health disparities are not a distraction. They are exactly where we must focus in order to understand what is going on. Senator Cassidy is a medical doctor. He should know better than to raise the harmful trope of Black people being genetically predisposed to be sicker than white people. This myth is not only untrue but racist and has no place in today's political discourse. Still, it's just one of many commonly held myths that pretend to explain why Black people experience

---

30 Louisiana Department of Health, Office of Public Health, "Addressing Disparities in Maternal and Child Health Outcomes for African Americans," September 2019, 2, https://ldh.la.gov/assets/docs/LegisReports/SR240HR294RS201992019.pdf.

31 James Doubek, "Louisiana Sen. Cassidy Addresses Racial Disparities in Coronavirus Deaths," NPR.org, April 7, 2020, https://www.npr.org/sections/coronavirus-live-updates/2020/04/07/828827346/louisiana-sen-cassidy-addresses-racial-disparities-in-coronavirus-deaths/.

higher death rates than white people both in general and specifically in maternal health and mortality. Focusing on genetics puts the blame on Black people themselves, discharging state responsibility for the problem.

This chapter will break down some of the myths surrounding Black maternal death rates to inform the senator and others who believe that death rates among Black people are mysterious at best and their own fault at worst. The good news—and bad news—is that we already know what is really causing these disgraceful health disparities. It's not genetics. It's not socioeconomic status. It's not culture. It's not class. It's not education. It's racism.

> Black people are more susceptible to dying in general and especially in pregnancy and childbirth due to systemic racism and inherent bias.

In this chapter, we'll explore why giving birth while Black in America is as dangerous if not more dangerous as it is in parts of the developing world.[32] To Raegan McDonald-Mosley, a former chief medical officer for the Planned Parenthood Federation of America, the data on Black maternal death rates clearly shows that "there's something inherently wrong with the system that's not valuing the lives of Black women equally to white women."[33] As Linda Villarosa, author of *Under the Skin: The Hidden Toll of Racism on American Lives*

---

32   Amy Roeder, "America Is Failing Its Black Mothers," *Harvard Magazine*, Winter 2019, https://www.hsph.harvard.edu/magazine/magazine_article/america-is-failing-its-black-mothers/.

33   Nina Martin and Renee Montagne, "Nothing Protects Black Women from Dying in Pregnancy and Childbirth," ProPublica with NPR News, December 7, 2017, https://www.propublica.org/article/nothing-protects-black-women-from-dying-in-pregnancy-and-childbirth.

and on the Health of Our Nation, eloquently puts it, "Yes, something is creating a health crisis, and that something is racism."[34]

The racism that causes so many Black people to die in pregnancy and childbirth comes from two directions. First, a racist society creates conditions that make Black people sicker than white people before they're pregnant, leading to worse health outcomes in pregnancy and childbirth. Second, a racist medical system treats Black people and their babies differently than white people and their babies, resulting in avoidable deaths. Until we address these two sectors of racism head on, forced pregnancy and childbirth due to abortion bans will affect Black people more than white people. That is, Black people will continue to be harmed and die at alarming rates. We must stop minimizing the issue. We must ask ourselves why, for "whatever reason," many in our government and our society are ignoring the inherent and systemic racism that is killing mothers, especially Black ones, in numbers that are not just disproportionately high but growing.

A RACIST MEDICAL SYSTEM TREATS BLACK PEOPLE AND THEIR BABIES DIFFERENTLY THAN WHITE PEOPLE AND THEIR BABIES, RESULTING IN AVOIDABLE DEATHS.

Genetics Aren't Destiny

Myth: "Black people are genetically different, making them prone to diseases that harm them and their babies in childbirth."

The idea that Black people are genetically different from others is a racist concept that dates back to slavery. According to the prevailing thinking at that time, enslaved Africans could work in the fields

---

34   Linda Villarosa, *Under the Skin: The Hidden Toll of Racism on American Lives and on the Health of Our Nation* (New York: Doubleday, 2022), 21. For an expansion of many of the topics in this chapter, see *Under the Skin*, for which this chapter is indebted.

longer due to not feeling pain the way white people did. Horrific experiments could be carried out on them without anesthesia due to the belief that enslaved people's nerve endings were less sensitive than white people's. In current times, when Black people go to the hospital concerned about pain, they are frequently dismissed, undermedicated, and undertreated compared to their white counterparts because of these perceived differences.

In other words, these false beliefs are not just historical. As Villarosa uncovers in her research, a 2015 study published in the *Proceedings of the National Academies of Science* showed that half of current medical students believe at least one untrue "fact" about Black bodies being fundamentally different from white bodies. The study also found that these beliefs led to treatment disparities such as withholding pain medications and even treatment itself.[35] This can be deadly when it comes to pregnancy and childbirth.

In truth, humans exhibit very little genetic variation, and the variation that does exist is very rarely defined by race. One Kaiser Research study showed that environment and other factors were twice as likely to cause premature death than genetics.[36] As Clarence Gravlee, associate professor at the University of Florida, explains, "The genes that influence skin color are distributed independently of genes that influence the risk for any particular disease. Given the heterogeneity of groups we call 'black' or 'white,' treating those categories as proxies for genetic variation almost always leads us astray."[37]

---

35   Kelly M. Hoffman, Sophie Trawalter et al., "Racial Bias in Pain Assessment and Treatment Recommendations, and False Beliefs about Biological Differences between Blacks and Whites," Proceedings of the National Academies of Science, March 1, 2016, https://www.pnas.org/doi/pdf/10.1073/pnas.1516047113.

36   Harry J. Heiman and Samantha Artiga, "Beyond Health Care: The Role of Social Determinants in Promoting Health and Health Equity," Kaiser Family Foundation Issue Brief, November 2015, https://policylink.org/sites/default/files/KFF-issue-brief-beyond-health-care.pdf.

37   Clarence Gravlee, "Racism, Not Genetics, Explains Why Black Americans Are Dying of COVID-19," Scientific American, June 7, 2020, https://blogs.scientificamerican.com/voices/racism-not-genetics-explains-why-black-americans-are-dying-of-covid-19/.

In other words, when people use genetics to explain away illnesses that are mostly environmental, they are usually wrong. These environmental conditions that are often ignored are called social determinants of health.

> Social determinants of health are the economic and social conditions outside of an individual's control that cause differences in health status.

Does a person have access to safe housing, healthy food, adequate medical care, and a society free of racism? If not, their health suffers. Racism, poverty, unsafe neighborhoods, unhealthy food, toxic environments, and so on are all social determinants of health that contribute to obesity, diabetes, high blood pressure, and other conditions that make pregnancy and childbirth more dangerous.

These social determinants of health will be explored more deeply in chapter 6 when we discuss reproductive justice, but for now understand that Black pregnant people are often sicker before they become pregnant because of their environments, not genetics. A huge part of that environment is living in a racist society. Living in a racist society puts extraordinary stress on Black bodies. Professor Arline Geronimus at the University of Michigan School of Public Health was a pioneer in research showing that racialized trauma is real. Centuries of discrimination and ongoing bias take their toll in what she calls *weathering*, a metaphor that expresses the accumulation of stress from racism in everyday life. Weathering due to the day-to-day stress of encounters with racist people and systems literally ages Black bodies the way wind and rain age a barn, breaking it down day by day, bit by bit.[38] In other words, one big reason Black people are sicker is because of premature aging brought on by racism.

That racism is a big part of the environment in which Black people live every day and can no longer be ignored. Until our politicians, doctors, and medical students learn this, Black people will continue to be harmed by this narrative that they are unfortunate victims of their bad genetic luck, with nothing to be done about their poor health.

Conflating Poverty and Race

Myth: "Black people are poorer than whites, so of course they have higher maternal death rates."

The belief that more Black mothers and their babies are dying because they're poorer than others is only partly true. Yes, poor people often have worse health. But people of color, especially Black people, have worse health outcomes even after correcting for class, education, and wealth.

A growing body of research supports this. One study found that men in Harlem, which is 96 percent Black, had shorter lifespans than men in Bangladesh, despite one-quarter of Harlem residents being middle or upper class and only 41 percent living below the poverty line.[39] Another study found that college-educated Black parents were twice as likely to lose their babies than similarly

COLLEGE-EDUCATED BLACK PARENTS WERE TWICE AS LIKELY TO LOSE THEIR BABIES THAN SIMILARLY EDUCATED WHITE PARENTS.

---

38 See Villarosa, *Under the Skin: The Hidden Toll of Racism on American Lives and on the Health of Our Nation*, pages 80–84 for a more detailed explanation of weathering and Geronimus's work.

39 C. McCord and H. P. Freeman, "Excess Mortality in Harlem," The New England Journal of Medicine 322, 3 (1990): 173–7. doi:10.1056/NEJM199001183220306.

educated white parents.[40] When maternal health data is corrected for wealth and education, the trends of alarmingly higher maternal Black death rates still hold. The Kaiser Family Foundation compiled data from the Centers for Disease Control and Prevention (CDC) that showed Black women with a college education or more had an over five times higher pregnancy-related mortality rate compared to white women with the same education. Black women with college or higher degrees were 1.6 times more likely to die from pregnancy-related causes than white women with less than a high school diploma.[41]

Weathering is a big part of the story, as money and status don't protect Black people from racism. Another reason socioeconomic status doesn't protect Black mothers or their babies is inherent and systemic racism in our healthcare system itself.

Racism in Healthcare

Myth: "We all have access to the same healthcare, so there's no inequality."

A while back, I entered an exam room to see my next patient, an African American woman. She had come with her friend, who was also Black, and when my patient saw me, she whispered to her friend in amazement, "She Black."

I said, "I heard that," to which she laughed and said, "But it's a good thing." We all nodded and smiled at one another. And I said, "I know."

---

40   Kenneth C. Schoendorf, Carol J. R. Hogue et al., "Mortality Among Infants of Black as Compared with White College-Educated Parents," *New England Journal of Medicine*, June 4, 1992, https://www.nejm.org/doi/full/10.1056/nejm199206043262303.

41   Samantha Artiga, Olivia Pham et al., "Racial Disparities in Maternal and Infant Health: An Overview," Kaiser Family Foundation, November 10, 2020, https://www.kff.org/report-section/racial-disparities-in-maternal-and-infant-health-an-overview-issue-brief/.

What we all knew is that the medical setting is an especially dangerous one for Black people. With only 2.5 percent of medical doctors being Black women and only 5 percent of US physicians being Black overall, it's rare for Black people to experience care with a Black doctor. But when they do, it matters. As Linda Villarosa explains:

> The majority of physicians are white and bring their individual biases to their work and, without being conscious of it, may have trouble humanizing and empathizing with people who are different from them. Research shows that Black patients benefit from having a Black health-care provider. A 2020 study showed that Black newborn babies in the United States are more likely to survive childbirth if they are cared for by Black doctors, but three times more likely than white babies to die when looked after by white doctors. The mortality rate for white babies was largely unaffected by the doctor's race.[42]

I often see this anecdotally in my practice. I once had a patient who told me "I just wanted to tell you that I am so glad that you were Black. I did not know who I was going to see. I thought I was going to be seeing some white man who would then go back to his family and talk about how he performed an abortion for another Black woman today. And I am just so happy that you are here. Honestly, I don't know what I would've done if I would've come here and it was a white doctor."

In other words, she felt that she wouldn't be seen as an individual by a white doctor but instead as someone representing her entire race. She was struggling with the weight of that responsibility—her concern

---

42   Villarosa, *Under the Skin*, 179–180.

over how she would be perceived based on the negative narrative she would have been contributing to. It was definitely weighing heavily on her, so much so that seeing me was a visible relief. I had taken this weight off her when I walked into the room.

That weight is a stress that other people don't have to deal with in a medical setting, so they don't understand it or even have any idea it exists. When she told me *I don't know what I would've done if it wasn't you who walked into the room,* it was clear to me that if I hadn't been Black, maybe she wouldn't have gotten the care she had come in to receive.

Were these feelings her own fault? Can we blame individual Black people for feeling this way? The mistrust, discomfort, and fear of judgment Black people feel in the medical setting is not a figment of their imagination.

History and data show us that my patient and others like her have every reason to be afraid.

The History of Reproductive Control

Myth: "Slavery and Jim Crow were a long time ago.
They don't have any effect on today's world."

To understand where we are today, we need to understand how we got here. During slavery, enslaved Black people were subjected to sustained, legalized sexual and reproductive violence. The US chattel slavery system treated Black women as breeding machines to meet the demands of the economic system built from their labor. Through arranged marriages, forced sexual encounters with other enslaved people, and rape by slave owners, enslaved Black women were subject to frequent sexual exploitation. They were not given a choice about who they had sexual relationships with, when, and the outcomes of those sexual relations. Then, women were blamed for these experiences as white male masters developed the "Jezebel" stereotype, minimizing Black women to passionate, hypersexual beings who wanted to engage in sexual acts with anyone and everyone.

> The trope of the hypersexualized Black woman endures and harms to this day.

In resistance to slavery and specifically sexual oppression, Black enslaved women often resorted to their own forms of abortion and contraception. They drew upon African folk remedies and Native American knowledge concerning local plant life to concoct medicines that would be shared and spread throughout the plantations. Southern physician E. M. Pendleton reported that plantation owners frequently complained about "the unnatural tendency in the African female population to destroy her offspring. Whole families of women ... fail to have any children."[43]

It's crucial to understand this history, because the end of slavery did not mean the end of racist stereotypes, attitudes, institutional racism, or the generational economic and emotional harm done to Black people in America. As researchers on Black reproductive health point out, "If past influences that have potentially shaped current outcomes are not taken into consideration, then public health efforts may neglect the impact of larger, contextual factors that affect health and contribute to inequities."[44]

---

43   E. M. Pendleton, MD, "Diseases of Hancock County," *Southern Medical and Surgical Journal*, ed. Paul F. Eve, MD (Augusta, Georgia: James McCafferty, 1849), 651.

44   Cynthia Prather et al., "Racism, African American Women, and Their Sexual and Reproductive Health: A Review of Historical and Contemporary Evidence and Implications for Health Equity," *Health Equity* 2, no. 1 (September 24, 2018), 249–259, doi:10.1089/heq.2017.0045, https://www. ncbi.nlm.nih.gov/pmc/articles/PMC6167003/.

In 1865, the Emancipation Proclamation granted freedom to enslaved Black people. However, Black codes and Jim Crow laws arose to continue to oppress and suppress the Black community. Sexual and reproductive abuses continued, such as rape laws only being enforced for white women, which were a direct threat to both Black women and men. Black people were victims of public lynching, many of which involved gang rape and genital mutilation.

It's crucial to remind ourselves that Jim Crow laws and Black codes did not formally end until President Lyndon Johnson signed the Civil Rights Act in 1964, that is, within the lifetime of many Black people alive today, their parents, and grandparents. This is not ancient history. And like slavery, the discrimination that these laws codified and the damaging results including stereotypes embedded in our culture from them did not end with the laws' demise. Racism persists, including attitudes about Black women and their reproduction. Proof of this is that even with Jim Crow laws gone, the American government kept up systemic racism in the form of forced sterilization and contraception in which the American medical system was fully complicit.

Forced Sterilization and Contraception

Myth: "Doctors and medical professionals are too educated to reflect the racism of society as a whole."

After emancipation, Black babies no longer furthered the economic gain of white Americans. Growing African American populations, which had been encouraged, were now perceived as a threat. Consequently, beginning in the early 1900s, another form of Black population control emerged. Eugenics programs spread across the nation to control Black population growth by way of coerced sterilizations.

Coinciding with the civil rights movement, a time in which the Black community was beginning to gain political autonomy, the government tried to restrict Black people's freedom through preventing Black women from becoming mothers. By 1970, Black women were sterilized at over twice the rate of white women: 9 per 1,000 for Black women as compared to 4.1 per 1,000 for white women.[45] One Princeton University study found that in 1970, 21 percent of married Black women had been sterilized.[46] Other minority groups, most notably Puerto Ricans and Native Americans, were also victims of racially motivated forced sterilizations, many in federally funded clinics. In 1965, it was estimated that one-third of Puerto Rican mothers between the age of twenty and forty-five were sterilized.[47] From the 1960s to '70s, one-quarter of Native American women were sterilized without their consent.[48]

State-sponsored eugenics were often forced on women of color either without their knowledge or with the threat that they'd lose their benefits or their children or they'd be subject to criminal prosecutions if they didn't comply. This contributed to the distrust of the medical system. While state-sponsored eugenics programs were halted in 1977, by then 100,000 to 150,000 poor, mostly Black women had been sterilized each year in the United States under federally funded programs.[49]

Adding to the distrust forced sterilization aroused, coerced use of long-term contraceptives to control minority populations was

45   Jennifer Nelson, *Women of Color and the Reproductive Rights Movement* (New York: NYU Press, 2003), 67.

46   Keeanga-Yamahtta Taylor, "How Black Feminists Defined Abortion Rights," *The New Yorker*, February 22, 2022, https://www.newyorker.com/news/essay/how-black-feminists-defined-abortion-rights.

47   Harriet B. Presser, "The Role of Sterilization in Controlling Puerto Rican Fertility," Population Studies 23, no. 3 (1969) 343–61, https://doi.org/10.2307/2172875.

48   Jane Lawrence, "The Indian Health Service and the Sterilization of Native American Women," *American Indian Quarterly* 24, no. 3 (2000), 400–19, http://www.jstor.org/stable/1185911.

49   Villarosa, *Under the Skin*, 38.

rampant through the 1970s. Like sterilization, many of these devices including IUDs and birth control implants were inserted without the understanding or consent of the recipients. They were also forced on women as conditions of receiving government benefits, keeping custody of existing children, or avoiding criminal prosecutions. While federal funds could often be used to implant the devices, these funds couldn't be used to remove them, leaving women unable to become pregnant if their minds or their circumstances changed.

Even the mainstream American contraceptive movement is being reevaluated in light of its racist history. For example, the legacy of "hero" and founder of Planned Parenthood, Margaret Sanger, is being reexamined due to her role in the eugenics movement. In July 2020, Planned Parenthood of Greater New York announced it would remove Sanger's name from their health center, explaining that "Margaret Sanger's concerns and advocacy for reproductive health have been clearly documented, but so too has her racist legacy. There is over-whelming evidence for Sanger's deep belief in eugenic ideology, which runs completely counter to our values ..."[50]

It's heartbreaking that contraception, an excellent tool that could help improve the lives of Black people and other people of color, was being used against them. It created lingering harm that to this day complicates individuals' relationship with the medical system and their own pursuit of better lives for themselves and their children. The false narrative of Black genocide then played on this shameful history, making the harm even greater.

---

50   "Planned Parenthood of Greater New York Announces Intent to Remove Margaret Sanger's Name from NYC Health Center," press release, July 21, 2020, https://www.plannedparenthood.org/planned-parenthood-greater-new-york/about/news/planned-parenthood-of-greater-new-york-announces-intent-to-remove-margaret-sangers-name-from-nyc-health-center; for more on Sanger, including a comprehensive list of sources, see, "Opposition Claims About Margaret Sanger," Planned Parenthood, April, 2021, https://www.plannedparenthood.org/uploads/filer_public/cc/2e/cc2e84f2-126f-41a5-a24b-43e093c47b2c/210414-sanger-opposition-claims-p01.pdf.

Black Genocide

Myth: "Abortion and contraception is a white-led conspiracy to eliminate the Black community."

While the government and medical community were working hand in hand to keep the Black community from reproducing, the anti-abortion movement was working to convince Black women this was reason enough to have their babies. Antiabortionists were joined by Black nationalists like Marcus Garvey, who believed in the "power of numbers" theory when it came to how Black people could obtain power in the United States. Birth control was explained as just another method of population control that was administered by the government to suppress the Black population.

Unfortunately, none of these groups actually helped people support children once they were born, and so they often suffered under the twin scourges of poverty and racism. As Shirley Chisholm, a Black congresswoman from Brooklyn in the 1970s, explains, "to label family planning and legal abortion programs 'genocide' is male rhetoric, for male ears … women know, and so do many men, that two or three children who are wanted and prepared for … will mean more for the future of the black and brown races … than any number of neglected, hungry, ill-housed, and ill-clothed youngsters."[51]

> The Black genocide trope is just another way to coerce and control Black women.

For antiabortion extremists, the forced birth of nonwhite people is just an inconvenience, a minor side effect. The real goal is for white women to have more babies. Black genocide narratives had the added

---

51   Dorothy Roberts, *Killing the Black Body* (New York: Vintage, 1998), 101.

"benefit" of keeping Black women poor and desperate, yet that was a secondary goal for the white nationalist aims of the antiabortion movement.

By exploiting Black religiosity and Black nationalism, the antiabortion movement was able to use the idea of Black genocide to capitalize on the internal dialogue among Black people about our ability to own our reproductive destinies. This discussion still comes into my medical practice in several forms. First, I see it in the confusion and stress of my patients as they grapple with the myriad conflicting forces that are trying to "protect" them from themselves, their own goals, and inner truths. Second, I see it in the hate I get from antiabortion forces. As I wrote in an amicus brief before the Supreme Court in the *Dobbs v. Jackson Women's Health* case that would ultimately overturn *Roe v. Wade*:

> FOR MANY OF MY PATIENTS, THESE CONFLICTING NARRATIVES OF HISTORICAL AND CURRENT REPRODUCTIVE CONTROL ARE EVER PRESENT.

> I have a trifecta of triggers for harassment: I'm Black, a woman, and I provide abortion care. Those are three ways that I am walking through the world and monitoring my spaces. I don't get called just "a baby-killer," I'm "a n****r baby-killer." I'm accused of "committing Black genocide." Those aren't things white abortion providers have yelled at them. And so, my level of vigilance is significantly heightened. But people need abortions, so I do what needs to be done to make sure abortion care is available to them.[52]

---

52   Thomas E. Dobbs, State Health Officer of the Mississippi Department of Health, et al., Petitioners, v. Jackson Women's Health Organization, et al., brief amicus curiae of Physicians for Reproductive Health, https://www.supremecourt.gov/DocketPDF/19/19-1392/192897/20210920113504270_210195a%20Amicus%20Brief%20for%20efiling.pdf, 11.

For many of my patients, these conflicting narratives of historical and current reproductive control are ever present. Whether prohibiting people from giving birth or coercing them into giving birth, they have the same effect: distrust of the medical community and their motives. When Black people enter the clinical setting, they encounter further racism that confirms their misgivings, as they are ignored or mistreated by racist doctors and staff. I tell my patients, *the racism you feel is real. It's difficult to call it out when you encounter it, but try. And when you can't, at least recognize to yourself that you're not overreacting or imagining things, because your life is literally at stake.*

Healthcare's First Steps

Myth: "Racism in healthcare might sometimes happen, but it's not that widespread."

By the summer of 2020, the data became impossible to ignore. The American Medical Association put out a statement that declared racism a public health threat in which the medical community was complicit:

> The AMA recognizes that racism negatively impacts and exacerbates health inequities among historically marginalized communities. Without systemic and structural-level change, health inequities will continue to exist, and the overall health of the nation will suffer … Declaring racism as an urgent public health threat is a step in the right direction toward advancing equity in medicine and public health, while creating pathways for truth, healing, and reconciliation.[53]

---

53   Kevin B. O'Reilly, "AMA: Racism Is a Threat to Public Health," American Medical Association, November 16, 2020, https://www.ama-assn.org/delivering-care/health-equity/ama-racism-threat-public-health.

In addition, the AMA board released a statement acknowledging that "racism and unconscious bias within medical research and healthcare delivery have caused and continue to cause harm to marginalized communities and society as a whole."

HISTORICAL AND CURRENT RACISM IN HEALTHCARE AND THE WORLD AS A WHOLE ISN'T IMAGINED.

They stated that "the AMA recognizes that worsening inequities, unequal access to care, and the disproportionately small number of Black physicians all have roots in past actions of the AMA … (including) more than a century of policies that excluded Black physicians."[54]

Historical and current racism in healthcare and the world as a whole isn't imagined. It's real, and it's a crisis. The first step to fixing it is to admit that it exists. The next step is to actually do something about it.

Society's Next Steps

Myth: "There's nothing we can do."

It's important that people understand the history and legacy of racism in this country and how it relates to maternal health. It's no longer enough to just say *I'm not racist.* We are asking people to be antiracist.

Antiracist means being committed to actively opposing racism and promoting racial tolerance.

When someone calls you racist, listen. You can't be a white person passively in America and not have racist ideology as part of who you are. Being antiracist is the ability to witness what somebody who doesn't

54   "AMA Board of Trustees Pledges Action against Racism, Police Brutality," American Medical Association, press release, June 7, 2020, https://www.ama-assn.org/press-center/press-releases/ama-board-trustees-pledges-action-against-racism-police-brutality.

look like you experiences when they're participating in institutions and systems and to try to find active ways to fix it. We can make lives better for all of society by actively learning about and challenging racist systems. A great place to start is by making sure that no one should have to be afraid of becoming a mother just because of the color of their skin.

TALKING ABOUT RACISM AND MATERNAL HEALTH

Myth: Racism has nothing to do with health.

Reality: "When I saw things from the point of view of the most vulnerable people, I started to understand all the barriers that some people face in accessing healthcare that I never even considered."

Myth: Diabetes, high blood pressure, and other diseases that hurt maternal health are higher in the Black community because of genetics.

Reality: "There are many reasons Black people have higher instances of some diseases, and the ones we can fix turn out to be the most important."

Myth: If we solve the problem of Black poverty, we solve the problem of high Black maternal mortality.

Reality: "Hearing about how Serena Williams almost died after her C-section because the healthcare professionals around her minimized her concerns made me realize that no amount of money can keep people safe from inherent, systemic racism."

Myth: Healthcare is color-blind.

Reality: "Healthcare professionals are just people, so of course they'll have the same weaknesses and prejudices of society as a whole."

Myth: Forced sterilization and coerced long-term contraception are things of the past.

Reality: "Knowing the history of eugenic programs and other abuses should make us more concerned about our government and healthcare system, not less."

Myth: Black Genocide is real.

Reality: "So many groups have their own agendas; it really takes time to untangle who is speaking for me and who is manipulating me for their own ends."

Myth: Fixing racism in healthcare is up to Black patients.

Reality: "It's exhausting to always be the one who has to speak up, especially at a doctor's office where I'm so vulnerable. The system has to be fixed from the inside."

Myth: There's nothing we can do about Black maternal death rates.

Reality: "When we stop blaming individual people and start looking at the conditions in which people are born, live, and work, we can find ways to stop people from dying."

CHAPTER FOUR

THE MYTH OF CAREFREE PREGNANCY AND CHILDBIRTH

Fifteen years ago, I was called into a hospital to save the life of a young mother of two who was twenty-two weeks pregnant. She was in the cardiac intensive care unit with a damaged and failing heart. During the pregnancy she developed an infection called endocarditis that generally is not lethal to a nonpregnant person. Unfortunately, the pregnancy was straining her heart, and traditional therapies were not working. Though she was dying, she declined abortion care as a lifesaving measure. Her strongly held religious beliefs influenced her decision to delay the only care that would keep her alive.

We explained to the woman, "You are dying, and we can help you live and return home to your children who need you."

The woman changed her mind after her health continued to worsen over a few days. After preparing her one day prior and securing the cardiac suite so that she could be placed on a mechanical device that helps pump blood from the lower chambers of the heart to the rest of the body during the procedure, the abortion was completed in five minutes. Her health began to improve immediately. The cardiology team and anesthesiologist looked on in amazement at how quickly her heart became stronger once the stress of the pregnancy was taken away. Two days after the abortion procedure, this dying woman went home to her family.

I am glad that she was able to choose her own life. No matter how hard our culture tries to project the picture of the smiling, glowing pregnant person who will breeze through and then recover from the tremendous changes the body undergoes to form and eventually birth a child, there will always be risk. Pregnant people should be able to decide for themselves how much risk they are willing to assume—not to have lawmakers or even physicians like me do it for them.

In order to assume that risk, people need to understand it. Myths and false narratives built up around pregnancy and childbirth make this understanding difficult. Our culture clings to a myth of idealized childbirth. Any deviation from this narrative is seen as proof that the individual is somehow deficient in morals, strength, or even "womanhood" itself. By this logic, a person seeking abortion care is the most uncaring, self-absorbed, awful person around—the opposite of the ideal, all-loving mother.

> OUR CULTURE CLINGS TO A MYTH OF IDEALIZED CHILDBIRTH. ANY DEVIATION FROM THIS NARRATIVE IS SEEN AS PROOF THAT THE INDIVIDUAL IS SOMEHOW DEFICIENT.

> The effortless, sentimental, glowing, selfless mother who breezes through pregnancy and childbirth with resolve and fortitude is lifted up in our society as a gold standard that then is used to shame anyone who does not conform to it.

An exploration of the discrepancies between the myth of idealized pregnancy and childbirth and people's lived experiences exposes some of the forces behind the myth:

Antiabortion advocates must downplay the sacrifice and danger to justify forced pregnancy and childbirth.

- Patriarchal society must perpetuate a rosy picture of motherhood to keep women in the home.

- White supremacist interests must make Black and Indigenous people and other people of color believe that a lack of access to healthcare and grossly uneven medical outcomes in maternal death are incidental to the abortion debate.

- Conservative and religious forces must vilify LGBTQ+ people to pass laws to prevent them from accessing the reproductive care they need.

I don't want to talk anyone out of pregnancy, childbirth, or parenting.

I've been blessed to share in joyful pregnancies and births as an obstetrician/gynecologist. But I also know that pregnancy and childbirth are serious business, and that they're more dangerous for people in historically marginalized groups than for white people. Passing any part of the process off as a minor inconvenience that "good" mothers should selflessly undertake and naturally succeed at is not just disingenuous; it's meant to shame and punish people who seek abortions or who give birth outside dominant narratives—especially people of color, disabled people, trans and nonbinary people, and the economically disadvantaged.

This chapter lays out some of the most harmful myths of idealized pregnancy and childbirth. It analyzes the reasons the myths exist. And it discusses how we can debunk them so that the risks we take to bear children (or to not bear them) are truly our own.

The Myth of the Carefree Pregnancy

Pregnancy is dangerous, even in the best of circumstances. Yet the myth that being pregnant and carrying a pregnancy to term is nine months of wonder and joy persists. Pregnant people are barraged with images of yoga on the beach, mommy facials, and smiling pregnant women in sunny rose gardens caressing their bellies. The remarkable similarity of pregnancy emoji from Google, Facebook, WhatsApp, and so on now include people of color and trans men, yet all are still smiling and holding their extended bellies with blissful smiles. Celebrities plaster their Instagram pages with sexy pregnancy pics. And the Bible tells us that "when a woman is giving birth, she has sorrow because her hour has come, but when she has delivered the baby, she no longer remembers the anguish, for joy that a human being has been born into the world" (John 16:21).

The myth that pregnancy is fully joyful or at worst just a temporary, minor inconvenience is not as dangerous as pregnancy and birth itself, yet it is still harmful. Anyone with varying experiences or feelings outside the dominant narrative is shamed and "othered." Not everyone is happy to be pregnant, and not every pregnancy turns out okay for the pregnant person or the fetus. In fact, early pregnancy is so fraught that 15 to 20 percent of pregnancies end in miscarriage.[55] Many people grieve the loss of these pregnancies in silence. They don't understand how common early pregnancy loss is. We don't talk about it due to societal norms that presume not carrying a pregnancy to term is a personal failure. Especially if someone's had multiple losses, the shame and stigma of being outside the norm can feel overwhelming. It can be exasperating for doctors like me on the front lines of reproductive health to see these risks and outcomes minimized as mere temporary inconveniences, meriting little or no regard.

> Pregnancy can and often does cause illness, lasting disease, disability, and death.

Common Conditions and Why They Matter

Many conditions that pregnancy brings on are so commonplace they are completely discounted: nausea, fatigue, sleeplessness, swelling, shortness of breath, cravings, dizziness, hormonal imbalance, back pain, hot flashes, heartburn, rashes, painfully stretched skin, frequent urination, fluid retention, and so on. Pregnant people are expected to continue to work and raise children through these conditions, often with little to no accommodation.

These conditions are often mild enough that a partnered person with support at home and a flexible, good-benefit, white-collar job can usually handle them. Pregnant people who fit this mold are considered the norm when pregnancy is discussed and when policy is created. For example, federal law mandates only twelve weeks unpaid family

---

55   Carla Dugas; Valori H. Slane, "Miscarriage," National Institutes of Health, June 27, 2022, https://www.ncbi.nlm.nih.gov/books/NBK532992/.

leave for pregnancy, birth, and childcare combined. Most lower-income people can't afford to take advantage of this unpaid leave, and strict eligibility requirements make it so that less than two-thirds of the US workforce is even eligible.[56] The people with service jobs who have to interact with customers all day or people with jobs on their feet like waitresses, nurses, or retail workers are often the least likely to be able to use their leave and also the people most likely to find it impossible to fight back "mild" nausea or other symptoms while also doing their jobs.

Many people who can't work through these conditions choose abortion rather than losing their livelihoods, especially if they already have children to support. We'll sometimes perform a surgical abortion without sedation because the person needs to go back to work that same night. Often, these people come to their abortion appointments with Family Leave Act papers from their employers. They've been working really hard at their jobs and also often at home raising existing children while they've been sick with pregnancy-induced conditions for weeks. By now, they're emotionally and psychologically exhausted. I'll give them three to four days off work if I can. The paperwork is often intrusive, so I try my best to fill it out as vaguely as possible to preserve the person's privacy, but I do have to mention that the leave is related to pregnancy and that a procedure happened. Some forms are so specific that they ask for diagnosis codes. I recently told a patient, "Legally, I don't have to tell your employer what your diagnosis was. I'm not going to answer that, and you don't have to either."

So when politicians or other people in a position of authority say a "normal" pregnancy is not a big deal, what they're really saying is that it's not a big deal for a person with resources to spare, family

56   Maya Rossin-Slater and Jenna Stearns, "The Economic Imperative of
      Enacting Paid Family Leave Across the United States," Washington Center
      for Equitable Growth, February 18, 2020, https://equitablegrowth.org/
      the-economic-imperative-of-enacting-paid-family-leave-across-the-united-states/#footnote-2.

support, and a white-collar, nonphysical, flexible job. For others, pregnancy can mean the difference between losing a job, a home, or even their existing children to the foster care system, a surprisingly common occurrence we'll discuss in the next chapter on parenting.

Bigger Problems Mean Bigger Disparities

Let's move on to the more grave yet not uncommon conditions that can develop, like preeclampsia (2–8 percent of pregnancies),[57] which can have no symptoms yet can cause damage to multiple organs; placenta previa (1 in 200 pregnancies),[58] which can cause severe bleeding and can be fatal; diastasis recti (60 percent of pregnancies),[59] which can cause bulging of the abdomen months if not years after giving birth; pelvic organ prolapse (25 percent of US women, mostly attributed to childbirth),[60] which can vary from annoying to needing surgical attention; miscarriage (15–20 percent of pregnancies),[61] which can cause mental distress and physical conditions from pain and bleeding to fatal hemorrhage; postpartum depression (10–20 percent of women);[62]

57   "Preeclampsia," March of Dimes, accessed September 30, 2022, https://www.marchofdimes. org/complications/preeclampsia.aspx#:~:text=Preeclampsia%20is%20a%20serious%20 health,before%2037%20weeks%20of%20pregnancy.

58   "Placenta Previa," March of Dimes, accessed September 30, 2022, https://www.marchofdimes. org/complications/placenta-previa.aspx#:~:text=Placenta%20previa%20happens%20in%20 about,other%20complications%20later%20in%20pregnancy.

59   Jorun Bakken Sperstad et al., "Lastasis Recti Abdominis During Pregnancy and 12 Months after Childbirth: Prevalence, Risk Factors and Report of Lumbopelvic Pain," *British Journal of Sports Medicine* 50, no. 17 (2016), https://www.ncbi.nlm.nih.gov/pmc/articles/PMC5013086/.

60   Ingrid Nygaard, Matthew D. Barber, Kathryn L. Burgio et al., "Prevalence of Symptomatic Pelvic Floor Disorders in US Women," *Journal of the American Medical Association* 300, no. 11 (2008): 1311-1316, https://pubmed.ncbi.nlm.nih.gov/18799443/.

61   Carla Dugas, Valori H. Slane, "Miscarriage," National Institutes of Health, June 27, 2022, https://www.ncbi.nlm.nih.gov/books/NBK532992/.

62   "Depression Among Women," Center for Disease Control, accessed September 30, 2022, https://www.cdc.gov/reproductivehealth/depression/index.htm#Postpartum.

gestational diabetes (6–9 percent of pregnancies);[63] high blood pressure (8–10 percent of pregnancies);[64] and more. Many of the conditions that occur for the first time during pregnancy, like diabetes and high blood pressure, often return after the pregnancy and become chronic later in life.

Numerous less-well-known conditions can land pregnant people in the hospital for extended stays. For example, nausea and vomiting in pregnancy is expected and tolerated by most people, but others develop a condition called hyperemesis gravidarum, which is debilitating nausea and vomiting. These people end up spending a significant amount of their pregnancy in and out of the hospital, which poses a risk to their jobs, children, and overall quality of life. Normal nausea during pregnancy generally will pass in the second trimester, but hyperemesis can go on well into the second trimester. It is just really a miserable condition to be in and affects at least sixty thousand pregnant Americans a year.[65]

HETERONORMATIVITY AND SYSTEMIC RACISM IN OUR SOCIETY AND IN OUR MEDICAL SYSTEM ... ALSO FACTOR INTO THE MANY WAYS THAT PREGNANCIES CAN HURT MARGINALIZED PEOPLE.

Sometimes, changes that happen in the body during pregnancy unmask heart conditions that people don't realize that they have, like cardiomyopathy, a defect in the heart muscle. Other times, people know of their condition before pregnancy, but they risk pregnancy anyway. People typically feel fine in the first trimester, but by the

---

63   "Diabetes During Pregnancy," Center for Disease Control, accessed September 30, 2022, https://www.cdc.gov/reproductivehealth/maternalinfanthealth/diabetes-during-pregnancy. htm#:~:text=develops%20during%20pregnancy.-,How%20Common%20Is%20Diabetes%20 During%20Pregnancy%3F,has%20increased%20in%20recent%20years.

64   "High Blood Pressure During Pregnancy," March of Dimes, accessed September 30, 2022, https://www.marchofdimes.org/complications/high-blood-pressure-during-pregnancy.aspx.

65   Pamela Paul, "There's No Such Thing as 'Just' Having a Baby," *New York Times*, June 20, 2022, A 17.

second trimester, they start to get elevated blood pressure and have trouble breathing, thus risking death. If these people continue their pregnancies, their heart can fail, and they can die.

All these conditions can happen to anyone, but they often most affect people who aren't in optimal health to begin with. Social determinants of health—safe housing, safe communities, and access to healthy food, transportation, outdoor space, clean water, and medical care—all affect people's health. For example, lack of nutritious food due to living in food deserts or lack of resources for proper nutrition can hurt health outcomes. Many lower-income people can't get to necessary health appointments because of subpar transportation or unreliable childcare. Lower-income people also often have employers who are not willing to work with them to provide time off for the frequent appointments that are required for a high-risk pregnancy, so they skip appointments, thus risking their health further. These people often can't afford to lose their jobs, as their insurance is tied to their employment, creating an added layer of stress and thus more illness. Heteronormativity and systemic racism in our society and in our medical system, which mirrors the implicit and explicit biases of healthcare professionals, also factor into the many ways that pregnancies can hurt marginalized people more than people who have the resources and entitled standing in society to maintain better health.

We need to address the root causes of poor maternal outcomes when we talk about who suffers the most risk from being pregnant. Only then can we understand that lack of abortion care hurts some people and communities more than others.

Myths around Mental Illness

Mental illness is another factor that can complicate a pregnancy. It's estimated that one in seven people will experience depression during pregnancy.[66] In addition, medications taken for a pregnant person's own mental health can harm a fetus, especially those taken for bipolar disorder. When I'm having this conversation with people, I tell them, "Your mental health is very important. If you have tried other medications and they have not worked for you and this particular medication, which is not safe in pregnancy, is working for you, then it's really important for you to think through what a decompensation of your medical condition means to continue the pregnancy. Would you be okay?" This is a decision that only the person themselves can make.

Mood and anxiety disorders are among the most common complications that occur in pregnancy. These disorders can extend beyond the perinatal period (a number of weeks immediately before and after birth) into the first twelve months after delivery. We hear about the baby blues, a common and temporary experience right after childbirth when a new parent may have sudden mood swings, feeling very happy, then very sad, or they may cry for no apparent reason. This is not considered a psychiatric illness. However, major depression and bipolar disorders can make the postpartum period very difficult if mistaken for the baby blues and left untreated. According to the American College of Obstetricians and Gynecologists, major depression "most often occurs in the first 3 months postpartum. [It] may also have started before pregnancy or begins during pregnancy, after weaning [the] baby or when [the] menstrual cycle resumes."[67] Bipolar

---

66 Rosemary Black, "Depression During Pregnancy: Millennials Suffer More than Previous Generation," PSYCOM, June 2022, https://www.psycom.net/depression-pregnancy.

67 "Summary of Perinatal Mental Health Conditions, Baby Blues, Unipolar/Major Depression, Bipolar Disorder," The American College of Obstetricians and Gynecologists, accessed September 30, 2022, https://www.acog.org/programs/perinatal-mental-health/summary-of-perinatal-mental-health-conditions.

disorder is generally diagnosed in the teens and early twenties, so some people can have a first onset in pregnancy or in the postpartum period.

It has been widely documented that the mental health of marginalized communities and their access to mental healthcare is not adequate, especially in the Black community. Issues such as the stigma of seeking mental health treatment, tropes of the "strong Black woman" who doesn't need help, the shortage of culturally sensitive and competent providers, and racism and bias in clinical settings and in the greater society all keep many from seeking the mental healthcare they need. When lack of economic resources, trauma, racism, oppression, and violence against Black people are entered into the equation, outcomes can be especially dire.

High-Risk Pregnancy

When a person wants to move forward with a high-risk pregnancy, we do everything we can to help them. We consult with a high-risk pregnancy specialist, and we plan. We make sure that the pregnant person delivers in a high acuity hospital that has the appropriate resources to sustain their life and health and that of the infant that will be delivered. If somebody lives in a rural community, their ability to get safely through a high-risk pregnancy and delivery when they have to travel becomes a big concern.

All the planning, pain, and risk of pregnancy and childbirth can be a temporary inconvenience for some people. For others, it can cost them their jobs, their homes, their savings, the welfare of their existing children, their mental health, and for some, their life. I want people to assume all this risk intentionally, to really understand what's at stake. Giving birth is not a mystical, mythical process that always turns out okay. I'm not trying to talk anyone out of pregnancy when I tell these stories. But when I tell somebody that they are highly likely to die or suffer long-lasting consequences if they continue a pregnancy, they should be able to decide for themselves what is best for them in the absence of a misguided narrative of birth that doesn't mesh with the reality of most pregnant people.

The Myth of the Joyful Birth

Childbirth is held up as a heroic act of bravery and courage— which it certainly is. However, it can also be so traumatic; it should not be entered into lightly or forced on anyone as it can lead to permanent disability or even death. The myth of the virtuous woman who endures this ordeal selflessly brings shame on the people who "fail." This allows the death of pregnant people to be discounted as a necessary evil, a small detour on the path to continuing the life of the child. America has a dismal track record on maternal death. As of this writing, America has the highest maternal death rate of any developed country, and that rate is increasing year over year.[68] Death rates for Black women are three to four times higher than for white people, even controlling for education and income.[69] Institutional and systemic racism is alive and well in America.

There are many factors that can lead to maternal deaths, many avoidable. The act of labor and pushing can exacerbate conditions of the heart and pulmonary systems for people who already have those chronic diseases. People with these conditions put their lives at significant risk as pregnancy progresses.

---

68   "Health and Health Care for Women of Reproductive Age: How the United States Compares with Other High-Income Countries," The Commonwealth Fund, issue brief, April 5, 2022, https://www.commonwealthfund.org/publications/issue-briefs/2022/apr/health-and-health-care-women-reproductive-age.

69   "Maternal Mortality Rates in the United States, 2020," Centers for Disease Control, accessed September 30, 2022, https://www.cdc.gov/nchs/data/hestat/maternal-mortality/2020/maternal-mortality-rates-2020.htm.

Long-term disability is another way that birth can be traumatic. Some years ago, I had a friend who was in labor for hours. The nurse could feel the head, but the baby wasn't coming. They moved her around, got her on all fours, all those things that people do to help the birth. Finally, her doctor determined that labor had been going on for too long and ordered a C-section. When they went in, they realized that the baby's head wasn't completely down; it was off to the side. That baby was never going to come out vaginally because it wasn't positioned to do so. My friend went to her postpartum visit complaining that her hip hurt, but her pain was dismissed as temporary. By the time she saw an orthopedic specialist a year later, she was told that the problem couldn't be surgically fixed. Too much time had passed since the initial injury. My friend now endures this silent disability for the rest of her life.

Another common occurrence during birth are tears of the cervix, vagina, vulva, anus, and even the urethra (the area you urinate from). Tears of the cervix can occur when a pregnant person begins to push when not fully dilated. Tears of the vagina can happen due to the breakdown of the tissues under the force of a prolonged second stage of labor when the head is not progressing down well. Vulvar and urethral tears can happen when the baby's head is delivered quickly, without a birth attendant to slowly guide the head out while supporting the surrounding structures. Anal tears are generally due to the use of a technique called an episiotomy. A small incision is made in the skin between the vaginal opening and the anus to allow more space for the delivery to occur. Sometimes that incision extends during birth to tear the muscles of the anus. These tears need to be repaired by stitches. I remember assisting with a birth where the baby delivered so quickly that the physician essentially caught it like a football. Upon examining the patient after delivering the placenta, we found tears along the urethra and vulva, down to her anus. I sewed everything back up. There are women who cannot hold their bowels and/or have urinary incontinence after childbirth for the rest of their lives.

A Note about C-Sections

Some people will choose a planned C-section to try to avoid the type of damage previously described. But C-sections carry risks, too, such as infection, hemorrhage, reactions to anesthesia, and more. In addition, multiple C-sections increase the risk of maternal death and disability. There is a condition called *placenta accreta* in which the placenta starts to grow into the scar in the uterus from a previous C-section. If that happens, then depending on how significant it is, the placenta does not separate completely. This causes a hemorrhage that can happen so quickly after the delivery of the placenta, a person could lose their entire blood volume in the matter of minutes. If it's really bad, it requires a removal of the uterus (a hysterectomy) in order to save the person's life.

I have experienced caring for patients with successful births after a C-section. I have also experienced a devastating uterine rupture and a baby that didn't make it. That harrowing experience gripped me emotionally for a long time.

The Morality of Mortality

I hope that outlining the risks of pregnancy and childbirth against the dominant narratives of happy, safe, joyous birth journeys will not just help people rationally decide on their own course of action but also give them some insight into the complexities physicians face every day.

It is not as simple as abortion opponents make it out to be when you are the one who has to take the life of the mother into consideration.

Once *Roe v. Wade* was overturned, my home state of Arizona enforced a near total ban on abortion. This law has one narrow exception—to save the life of the pregnant person. What does this even mean? Does the pregnant person have to be imminently dying? Or just highly likely to die? How likely? Fifty percent? Eighty? Ninety? In this post-*Roe* America, the individual abortion provider and their attorneys have to make that call.

I had to consider what I would do. Instead of deciding on a case-by-case basis whether I would perform an abortion or not, my goal was to run through different scenarios with my legal team and have them tell me what they feel my risk is based on each scenario. As of the writing of

WE NEED TO ASK OURSELVES AS A SOCIETY IF WE CARE, AND IF WE DON'T, WE NEED TO UNDERSTAND WHY.

this chapter, I stopped all abortion care in my clinic. Clarity around how the state expected compliance with the abortion ban was needed.

The laws are so badly written and so unclear, it's really much safer for physicians to just refuse to perform abortions at all. Some providers made the choice not to resume providing abortion care during the moment of uncertainty immediately after the Supreme Court decision that ended *Roe*. When this becomes the norm, the woman dying in the cardiac care ward at the start of this chapter will likely die. We need to ask ourselves as a society if we care, and if we don't, we need to understand why.

TALKING ABOUT PREGNANCY AND CHILDBIRTH

Myth: Being pregnant is just a minor inconvenience.

Reality: "My boss told me that she just 'powered through' her back pain when she was pregnant, but she just sits at a desk all day while I have to be on my feet. It's not the same. I need to talk to her again to get some accommodations, because this is too hard."

Myth: Complications during pregnancy and childbirth are rare.

Reality: "I know I'm lucky to have gotten through my pregnancy without any complications because a lot can and does go wrong."

Myth: Forcing pregnant people to give birth is not a big deal.

Reality: "After twenty-three hours of unsuccessful back labor, I had a C-section that led to life-endangering hemorrhaging. Now, I can't stop thinking about how close my other two children came to growing up without a mother."

Myth: The dangers of pregnancy and childbirth are the same for all people.

Reality: "Once I ended up on six weeks of doctor-ordered bed rest, I started thinking for the first time about all the people who don't have a partner or the financial resources to get them through an unexpected hardship like this."

Myth: Even if abortion is mostly banned, people who still need abortion intervention in dangerous situations will be able to get it.

Reality: "I really need to think about what will happen if my heart condition gets bad during my pregnancy. All those confusing rules means my doctors might be unwilling or unable to intervene."

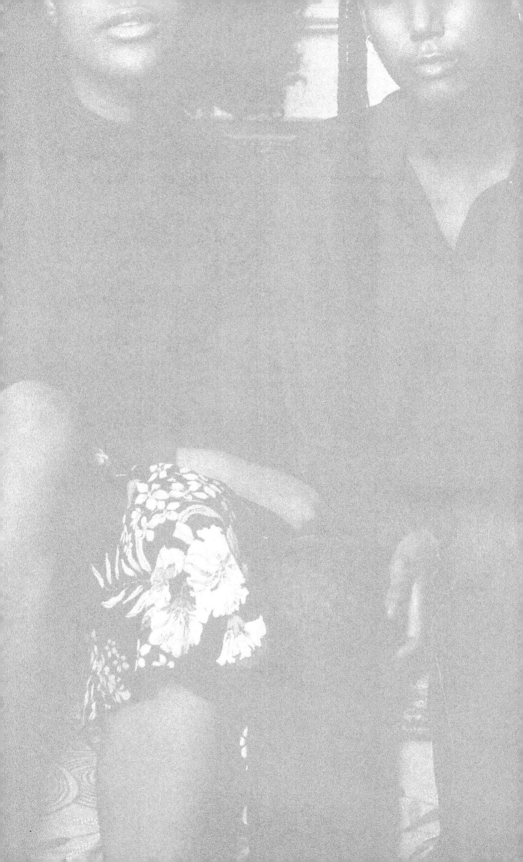

CHAPTER FIVE

MYTHS OF MOTHERHOOD AND PARENTING

A Reality Check

Who counts as a mother and who doesn't?

The Supreme Court opinion in *Dobbs v. Jackson Women's Health* that reversed *Roe v. Wade* gives us some clues as to who matters and who doesn't when we talk about mothers. In his majority opinion, Alito argues that "modern developments" make past burdens of motherhood obsolete. These developments include "attitudes about the pregnancy of unmarried women" that have "changed drastically"; the existence of state laws that "ban discrimination on the basis of pregnancy"; and the fact that the costs of medical care associated with pregnancy are "covered by insurance or government assistance." He also brings up safe-haven laws that allow mothers to "drop off" babies for adoption with "little reason to fear" and federally mandated family leave policies that protect jobs. In Alito's imagined world, then, mothers are respected by society, have secure jobs, adequate health insurance, and government-mandated time off to raise their families.[70]

The reality for many people looks quite different:

- **On single mothers:** Although one in three children in America grow up in single-parent households,[71] their mothers are still lacking their most important need: affordable childcare. There are many reasons for this, but one is that single mothers are still held in contempt by society. The 2022 Republican candidate for Ohio Senate, J. D. Vance, expressed this sentiment succinctly when he tweeted in April 2021 that "universal day care is class war against normal people."[72] A few months later, he won his senate race.

- **On discrimination at work:** The National Partnership for Women & Families found that "women in all industries, across race and ethnicity, and in every state, continue to experience pregnancy discrimination in the workplace." However, between 2011 and 2015, Black women filed nearly 30 percent of all pregnancy discrimination charges with the Equal Employment Opportunity Commission, even though they made up only 14 percent of women in the workforce ages sixteen to fifty-four.[73]

---

70 Dobbs, State Health Officer of the Mississippi Department of Health, et al. V. Jackson Women's Health Organization et al., June 2022, https://www.supremecourt.gov/opinions/21pdf/19-1392_6j37.pdf.

71 "Child Well-Being in Single-Parent Families," The Annie E. Casey Foundation, August 1, 2022, https://www.aecf.org/blog/child-well-being-in-single-parent-families?gclid=Cj0KCQiAg_KbB-hDLARIsANx7wAzo04IzXUdy0f6PaDtUAjSVEOP6zTaQMIuRaX81uv_2eA6GZ5rKvGkaAkmEEALw_wcB.

72 J. D. Vance, Twitter post, April 29, 2021, 9:41 a.m., https://twitter.com/JDVance1/status/1387763955557445640?s=20.

73 "By the Numbers: Women Continue to Face Pregnancy Discrimination in the Workplace," National Foundation for Women & Families, October 2016, https://www.nationalpartnership.org/our-work/resources/economic-justice/pregnancy-discrimination/by-the-numbers-women-continue-to-face-pregnancy-discrimination-in-the-workplace.pdf.

- **On access to comprehensive health insurance:** In April 2020, researchers found that in periods during and after pregnancy, "all categories of racial–ethnic minority women experienced higher rates of uninsurance than white non-Hispanic women." The numbers were significant: 75.3 percent of white, non-Hispanic women were continually insured compared to 55.4 percent of Black, non-Hispanic women, 49.9 percent of Indigenous women, and 20.5 percent of Latine, Spanish-speaking women.[74] As I see in my medical practice every day, even women who have insurance are often saddled with big copays and other significant unmet medical costs.

- **On family leave:** The federal Family and Medical Leave Act guarantees twelve weeks of *unpaid* family leave, yet only one in four workers have paid family leave.[75] Not surprisingly, these workers tend to have higher-paying jobs.[76] In addition, Black and Latine workers had significantly less access to paid leave through their employers or through government programs than their non-Hispanic white and Asian counterparts.[77]

- **On trans, nonbinary, and nonheterosexual parenthood:** Alito went out of his way to say that the *Dobbs* ruling doesn't affect other rights, but Clarence Thomas, in his concurring opinion, stated that the court should "reconsider" its opinion

---

74 Jamie R. Daw et al., "Racial and Ethnic Disparities in Perinatal Insurance Coverage." *Obstetrics and Gynecology* 135, no. 4 (2020): 917–924, doi:10.1097/AOG.0000000000003728, https://www.ncbi.nlm.nih.gov/pmc/articles/PMC7098441/.

75 "Paid Leave in the U.S.," Women's Health Policy, Kaiser Family Foundation, December 17, 2021, https://www.kff.org/womens-health-policy/fact-sheet/paid-leave-in-u-s/.

76 US Bureau of Labor Statistics, "Employee Benefits Survey," accessed June 8, 2022, https://www.bls.gov/ncs/ebs/.

77 Julia M. Goodman et al., "Racial/Ethnic Inequities in Paid Parental Leave Access," *Health Equity* 5, no. 1 (October 13, 2021): 738–749, doi:10.1089/heq.2021.0001, https://www.ncbi.nlm.nih.gov/pmc/articles/PMC8665807/.

on the right to contraception and same-sex marriage.[78] In this chapter, I'll often address the dominant heteronormative narrative, acknowledging that trans and nonbinary people experience pregnancy, childbirth, and parenting under these same conditions and that their rights and issues are either ignored (as by Alito) or directly threatened (as by Thomas).

As all this data makes clear, when Justice Alito and his supporters laid out the argument that our society and our law adequately support mothers, they were talking about a specific sort of mother—a white,

THEY WERE TALKING ABOUT A SPECIFIC SORT OF MOTHER—A WHITE, MARRIED ONE WITH GOOD HEALTH INSURANCE AND A FLEXIBLE, WHITE-COLLAR JOB.

married one with good health insurance and a flexible, white-collar job. That Alito centers this narrative isn't surprising. We are barraged with images of this ideal mother on television, in movies, and on social media. This woman sails through motherhood with the full support of society as part of a middle-class, heterosexual, nuclear family. Anyone who does not conform to this myth is not only left out of the conversation, but they are also marginalized, shamed, and punished.

Myth-Building from All Sides

Centering this imagined mother is not just the work of conservative justices, senators, and society. As was discussed in chapter 1, the mainstream women's movement and specifically the pro-choice movement is also guilty of focusing the conversation about motherhood on white ciswomen. We'll look more at the history of the movement and how

---

78   Dobbs, State Health Officer of the Mississippi Department of Health, et al. V. Jackson Women's Health Organization et al., (Thomas concurring) 3, https://www.supremecourt.gov/opinions/21pdf/19-1392_6j37.pdf.

it left people outside its narrative behind in chapter 6, but for now, it's important to point out that the issues deemed important to the mainstream women's rights movement are often based on assumptions that apply only to a small subset of privileged women, and its goals are primarily to increase that privilege. Again, the only way to fix this obsession on one type of mother is to look outside the narrow conversation of abortion rights and what it means to be pro-choice and instead focus on human rights and what it means to be proabortion. That is, it's time to talk about the right of all people to have safe environments in which to raise children or not have them as they see fit.

Why We Leave People Out

Why do we want to deny any person outside the good-mother narrative the abortion care they seek and then withhold help and empathy when they do raise children? What good is there in shaming others? In making their lives difficult if not impossible?

A racist, patriarchal society has an interest in upholding their vision of a society in where the people who have been pushed to the margins "rightly" suffer in poverty and women are denied autonomy over their lives.

Antiabortion advocates who claim to be pro-life can justify not supporting children after they're born based on prejudice against nontraditional families who they feel deserve their fate for not conforming to the "norm."

> They're not just deciding which mothers count and which do not, but they are deciding who can be a family and who cannot.

By punishing the people outside the myth of "traditional" motherhood, they quite literally keep them in their places, creating a cycle of misery. This conservative image of a heteronormative, white family justifies withholding the resources that would allow anyone outside the narrative to thrive. Single, Black, transgender, nonbinary, gay, lesbian, disabled, or low-income people get left behind as unworthy. We don't have universal healthcare, sufficient paid family leave, support for children with special needs, or maternity leave because the people who need them are deemed individually lacking by not fitting the ideal. We pass burdensome rules that force people to continue pregnancies and bring children into the world, but we withhold the support systems to help sustain them. Then we say it's the mother's fault that she's poor or "failing," which leads to shame, and the cycle continues.

> Parenting is not easy. Parenting outside the dominant paradigm can be close to impossible.

The Myth of Joyful Motherhood

Many people embrace motherhood and experience great joy in it. But not all. That motherhood might not bring joy is so unthinkable, that for many, it's out of the realm of imagination. Women who don't want children are often lectured on their "ticking clocks." They are denied hysterectomies that are at times medically necessary because medical professionals elevate the role of bearing children as so essential to a woman's essence, it's inconceivable that a person could truly want to be child-free. And, of course, they are often denied abortion care. Even women's groups often leave these women out, as their existence is so foreign to the ideal. As the Republican candidate for Arizona governor expressed in a tweet celebrating the fall of *Roe*, "A new chapter of Life has begun. A chapter where we help women become the Mothers they are meant to be. Thank you, God."[79]

When people who already have children want to control the size of families, they also experience shaming. Many mothers who come

> MANY MOTHERS WHO COME TO ME FOR ABORTIONS FEEL THE NEED TO STRESS TO ME THAT THEY LOVE THEIR CHILDREN, BUT THEY JUST CAN'T SUPPORT ANOTHER CHILD.

to me for abortions feel the need to stress to me that they love their children, but they just can't support another child at this moment in their lives. I can feel in their words the need to prove themselves as still worthy of the "loving mother" ideal. After all, if one or two children bring joy, then more babies should bring more joy. I usually tell them that the decision to have an abortion is not a tragedy or proof that they're a bad mother. It is the rational decision of a good mother supporting the children she already has. Abortion is just one of the decisions in a spectrum of decisions that pregnant people make. I remind them that most people who have abortions already have children, so they understand how important parenting is. Unfortunately, the myth of always-joyous motherhood does not have a place for these women. Remember, one in four women will have an abortion. That these people

---

79   Kari Lake, Tweet, June 24, 2022, @KariLake, https://twitter.com/karilake/status/15403654747219 76321?lang=en.

remain silent in their shame furthers the erasure of anyone outside the narrative of the happy, forever-selfless mother.

If happy child-free people and happy mothers with limited families are suspect, then unhappy mothers are considered downright deviant. But this is not reality. Up to one in five women will suffer from a postpartum mental health disorder like postpartum depression after childbirth. That we can't talk about this is again tied up with the shame of betraying the myth that motherhood is blissful. Mental health professionals and even celebrity mothers are beginning to break down these barriers. Gwyneth Paltrow confessed her postpartum depression in a *Good Housekeeping* interview, saying, "I couldn't access my heart. I couldn't access my emotions. I couldn't connect … I just thought it meant I was a terrible mother and a terrible person." That even a wealthy, educated feminist would think she was unworthy for feeling this way shows the prevalence and deep hold of the myth that all mothers must be joyous.

Mothering while Poor

There is no mother more outside the ideal than the infamous "welfare mother." To the public imagination, she is a conniving, manipulative, lazy, loose woman who abuses the welfare system as a way of avoiding work. Also, she's usually thought of as Black, even though the majority of people on welfare are white. That this imaginary person should be rewarded with "free" money from the government arouses anger, allowing the state to punish, shame, police, and control her as they see fit.

I see this kind of thinking at work in my home county of Maricopa, which includes Phoenix, where my clinic is located. Here, parenting while poor is so routinely punished, it's almost outside the realm of imagination. In Arizona, almost four out of every ten children will experience at least one Department of Child Services investigation during their childhoods. For Black children, that number increases to almost seven out of every ten children. And what happens to these children?

> Black children in Arizona are four times as likely to be placed into the foster care system by the state than their white peers.

In Arizona, only 8 percent of children enter the foster care system because they are being physically or sexually abused. Ninety-two percent of our children end up in foster care because of what is labeled "neglect." That might mean that a family doesn't have the ability to purchase clean diapers or healthy food. It could mean that they don't have access to medical care when it's needed due to insurance or transportation issues. In other words, the state is taking children away from their families because they are too poor to meet their physical, medical, or nutritional needs.

> The state is saying that poor people do not have the right to be mothers, especially if they're Black.

Then, when we further take away these families' access to abortion care, we are basically setting them up for more failure by forcing them to parent in impossible conditions.

How could we instead help these families? Many states use block grant money given to them from the federal government to directly support families through public assistance programs. In Arizona, we do this through what is called TANF—Temporary Assistance for Needy Families. Yet in Arizona, only six out of one hundred children who live in poverty get direct TANF benefits. Two-thirds of our block grant federal money goes to the Department of Child Services (DCS) system to support foster care and DCS investigations. So the money that is supposed to help families living in poverty with their basic needs is instead used to maintain the system that actively investigates and then dismantles these same families.

Families who do manage to get benefits are faced with time limits, punishments for having additional children, and strict adherence to rules and guidelines that are often impossible to meet. As Zaida Dedolph from the Children's Action Alliance points out, "We could make TANF, Medicare, and CHIP more available and more afford-able. We could change how we run our child welfare systems to best use those dollars in different ways. We could prioritize things like nutrition assistance at the state level, so that we're not as subject to federal funding for these programs. We could cut out the red tape and not make people jump through hoops to prove that they deserve to eat and have a place to live. But we don't. And until all of those things happen, we're going to be a hostile place for children and families."

Of course, she doesn't mean all children and families. She means children and families who are poor, especially those who are Black. She means children and families who fall outside the myth of the ideal and thus are considered unworthy of our help.

The Myth of Happy Adoptions

During oral arguments in December 2021 for *Dobbs v. Jackson Women's Health Organization*, Supreme Court Justice Amy Coney Barrett suggested that safe-haven laws and the availability of adoption in general relieved women of the burden of motherhood. Since a woman could just give her baby up for adoption, she mused, then forced parenting wasn't an issue. Alito followed this line of thinking in his final opinion overturning *Roe v. Wade* when he wrote that "a woman who puts her newborn up for adoption today has little reason to fear that the baby will not find a suitable home." Like the happy narratives around pregnancy, birth, and parenting, adoption is also held up as a moral, loving, and courageous decision sure to bring happiness to all involved.

Adoption is not the panacea the justices imagine. I have had patients who have had both abortions and adoptions, and what haunts them the most is the adoption. Worrying about the child that they gave away is what keeps them up at night, not the abortion that they had. That child is in the world. They're thinking about it. It's distressing. In other words, they are still parents, but someone else is raising their child. Their experience strengthened their belief that the abortion was the better choice for their mental health. Indeed, the landmark book *The Turnaway Study* that followed one thousand women for ten years, half who had abortions and half who were turned away shows that "the women who had the hardest time emotionally were those who placed their children up for adoption."

ADOPTION IS NOT THE PANACEA THE JUSTICES IMAGINE.

Rebecca Todd Peters, in her book *Trust Women: A Christian Argument for Reproductive Justice*, argues that difficulty with adoption arises because of a person's "intuitive recognition of the moral distinction between the (fetus) and the newborn baby." In other words, once a child has been born, it has become an actual person, so giving it up feels significantly different from aborting a fetus.

Giving a child up for adoption isn't the rosy picture the justices paint for the adopted child either. Adopted children often struggle with issues of abandonment. The issues that arise from interracial adoption, especially of Black and other children of color raised in white families, are especially acute. Questions about identity cause emotional issues, as adoption can lead to erasure of culture and identity for Indigenous people and other people of color. Adoption is often part of a white-savior narrative in which a white parent "rescues" a child from their "bad" environment. This environment could be a minority community, an LGBTQ+ household, or just an impoverished family in a world in which being poor means you're not a suitable parent. Add to all this the many children who don't get adopted at all, and a more nuanced picture of adoption arises. Currently, there are over four hundred thousand children in the foster care system in which the average child spends two years. Adoptee rights organizations expose these often-buried truths that don't fit the prevailing narrative, but their voices are clearly not being heard by those in power.

The Myths around People with Disabilities

It is estimated that one in four women in the United States live with a disability, and 10–12 percent of women of childbearing age have a disability. People with disabilities have sex, experience pregnancy, and give birth. Many can have healthy pregnancy outcomes when accommodations are tailored to their specific disability. Parenting with a disability requires a wide variety of adaptive strategies to make caring for infants and toddlers easier, including home modifications, using or creating accessible baby-care equipment, accessing support and information, and getting support from other people. Ableism (discrimination in favor of able-bodied people) is very widespread among our dominant patriarchal heteronormative culture and can be the gateway to other forms of prejudice toward people with disabilities. Harmful narratives regarding the bodies and minds of people with disabilities often leave them labeled deviant, unproductive, and/ or disposable.

For example, I've been part of a care team for a paraplegic pregnant person. They, too, get to be parents. This is a very important part of this conversation about what families look like. The reproductive capacity of everyone matters. Disabled people need to have families, sex, birth control, obstetrical care, and abortions. And yet, I've seen people not being able to get into the doctor's office with their wheelchair, people not being able to be positioned on the gynecology exam table, and healthcare workers not having conversations with people around issues of sex and contraception because they assume people with disabilities don't have sex. Opening our minds to every kind of family and every kind of mother is the first step to addressing these issues. To do this, we need to destroy the myth of who counts as a mother and who does not. All mothering is hard and deserves to be supported; mothering while disabled deserves support, too, so all can thrive. The right to bear children, or not bear children, and parent children in safe and sustainable communities does not change because an individual has a disability.

The other side of the disability conversation concerns children with special needs. The pro-life movement often points to the disability community when introducing legislation like the Arizona ban on abortion care for fetal genetic abnormalities that was signed into law in 2021. Supporters of the ban "insisted the legislation would protect Arizona's most vulnerable, preventing 'modern day eugenics' by ensuring equal treatment for babies with genetic conditions." This rhetoric echoes the disability community's call for all people to be valued. Unfortunately, the bill provides no help to these children or their families once they are born.

Families can find so much joy in caring for their member with a disability. However, the usual challenges of parenting are compounded for parents and primary caregivers of children with special needs. Some challenges include learning about the disability; researching, locating and accessing treatments and resources; coping with the demands of caring for an individual with a disability mentally and physically; coordinating appointments with medical providers, therapists, advocates, and school personnel; advocating for appropriate interventions, accommodations, or placements at school; and paying for the many treatments and interventions that are not covered by health insurance or the school system. A broad support system for the child and for the parents is needed.

The only person who can decide what they and their family can handle is the person who is pregnant. I remember reading a Facebook group thread discussing abortions for fetal diagnoses (a.k.a. genetic abnormalities). The conversation consisted of people talking about how their children with disabilities are the lights of their families. While I believed these people were sincere in their statements, I also thought, *There are several thousand women in this group. I bet there's someone who had an abortion for a fetal diagnosis.* However, this thread went on for a couple of days before I decided to step into the gap as an abortion provider who has cared for people terminating pregnancies for fetal genetic diagnosis like Down syndrome and also for abnormalities that were not compatible with life. I pointed out that the average person who would give birth to a child with special needs likely does not have the resources to care for that child, and many are already struggling. There are choices they might need to make for their family in a society

THE ONLY PERSON WHO CAN DECIDE WHAT THEY AND THEIR FAMILY CAN HANDLE IS THE PERSON WHO IS PREGNANT.

that doesn't provide enough support. My commentary was not well received, which highlighted for me how it wasn't even okay to say that it was hard to raise a child with special needs.

If you were in that Facebook group, reading that thread, and you only saw how wonderful it was, would you then step in and say, *That's not been my experience?* After my statements someone eventually spoke of their decision to have an abortion for a fetal genetic diagnosis. As long as we continue the myth of everything-is-rosy motherhood, we erase the existence of families that need substantial help or are having extreme difficulty coping with raising a child with disabilities.

Like so many other issues around motherhood, when the rights of the disabled are seen through the lens of reproductive justice, the conversation shifts. It's no longer about judging the choices individual people make to have or not have an abortion, but it's about society supporting people in their choices. We need to acknowledge the existence of people who don't have the resources to raise a child with a disability, and we need to support them. To do that, we can't be afraid to talk about them. As long as the myth that all is well dominates, that conversation is not permitted to happen. Talking about a diverse range of families is the only way to create space, equality, and self-determination for all. People with disabilities and their families are neither tragedies nor heroes. They are people with specific needs that deserve support, and to get that, we must acknowledge they exist as real people with real problems.

Queer, Trans, and Nonbinary Parents

Queer, trans, and nonbinary people also suffer when we center the experiences of white, married ciswomen. People whose gender identity does not match the gender assigned at birth or who reject heteronormative relationships often face considerable barriers accessing healthcare and government services to support their families.

Adoption is often difficult for anyone outside the normative family. Although same-sex adoption is currently legal in all fifty states, religious and foreign adoption agencies routinely deny these couples access. Even when having children themselves, same-sex couples often feel the need to take the extra step of having the nonbirthing parent formally adopt their children, adding extra protection in case their family is in the future deemed illegitimate. As one same-sex parent explained to *Rolling Stone* magazine, "Most dads cut their kids' umbilical cords, and then never have to think about it again ... I have to explain to my kid why we are going to the courthouse so that I could claim my rights as her parent." Now that Supreme Court Justice Clarence Thomas has indicated his view that same-sex marriage is up for review in his concurrence in the *Dobbs v. Jackson Women's Health Organization* decision eradicating *Roe*, this fear has become more dire.

Access to artificial reproductive technologies is also often difficult for transgender and queer people. This includes the ability to access in vitro fertilization and other ways to give birth with the help of modern medicine that were originally developed to give infertile or low fertility heterosexual married couples children. It takes effort and intention to expand access. Instead, as one study pointed out, although 25 percent of fertility clinic users in urban areas identify as LGBTQ+, these people "experience heteronormative and CIS normative assumptions at fertility clinics" due to a "lack of education and training." This "reinforces existing structures and forms of power and privilege where dominant groups are 'empowered to nurture and reproduce, while others are disempowered.'"

Reproductive Justice Counts
All Birthing People

Let's not erase Black, disabled, unmarried, Indigenous, poor, or LGBTQ+ or people of color when we talk about mothers. Let's instead center them in our conversation. Centering looks like using the term *parent* or *birthing person* instead of *mother* to illuminate that trans men and nonbinary people give birth. Let's look at the myths of motherhood and who counts and who doesn't through the lens of reproductive justice to better account for what's really happening on the ground. The government is central to creating the conditions that help people to live and thrive, and until we make sure they do that for all people, not just some, then we can't really say that we support birthing people and families. When we force people to continue pregnancies and bring children into the world without guaranteeing any of the support systems to help sustain them, or even considering their needs at all, we are creating conditions of misery. It's important to note, though, that we can't just blame the government. Our politicians reflect our society. We must be aware of our own prejudices about who counts and who doesn't before we can begin to change things for the better.

TALKING ABOUT PARENTING

Myth: Parents and families are supported by the social safety net.

Reality: "I didn't realize how many hoops people have to jump through to get the benefits they need to keep their families safe and how hard so many of those conditions are to meet. Now I understand why so many children are living in poverty."

Myth: People who have abortions don't want to be parents.

Reality: "I love being a mother, and that's why I had an abortion. It's the best choice for the two children I already have. Learning that 60 percent of people who get abortions are already parents made me understand I wasn't alone."

Myth: All people welcome parenthood and in it find their ultimate joy.

Reality: "We have to talk more about postpartum depression and about feelings of being overwhelmed by parenthood, or else people will think that they're alone, when really, all of us struggle."

Myth: Adoption is an alternative to abortion.

Reality: "I was either going to have my child and keep it or have an abortion. There's no way I would ever have been able to give up to a stranger a child that I'd held in my arms."

Myth: Families should look a certain way, and if they don't, society shouldn't have to support them.

Reality: "Single mothers, gay parents, trans parents—there are so many kinds of families out there. Our social policies ought to support them, and it's our responsibility as citizens to understand the core reasons why they don't."

CHAPTER SIX

REPRODUCTIVE JUSTICE

How to Move Beyond the "Choice" Narrative

A few months before *Roe v. Wade* was overturned by the Supreme Court, I hired a young Black woman to work in my clinic. During her first week with us, my staff and I were talking about an interview that I had done. The new staffer listened for a while, and then she stopped us. Sheepishly, she said, "I have a question. What is *Roe v. Wade?*"

I said to her, "Do not even be embarrassed, because you just confirmed what I've been trying to tell advocates—that the average person does not understand what we're talking about when we talk about *Roe*." Abstract conversations about the constitutional right to privacy and bodily autonomy, while valid, don't touch people where they live until they actually need abortion care. In states hostile to abortion access, that's often too late.

Meanwhile, the antiabortion movement has been waging a war over "dead babies," "God's will," "Black genocide," and "murder." They use emotional, heated rhetoric that activates their base, enabling them to take over statehouses and enact onerous restrictions even though over 70 percent of people in America support abortion rights and one in four American women of reproductive age will get an abortion before the age of forty-five. They control the conversation because they have figured something out the pro-choice side hasn't: the message has to relate to everyday people in their everyday lives, not just when they find themselves with an unexpected or dangerous pregnancy.

Now that *Roe* has fallen, not much has changed. Just as with *Roe*, everyone is earnestly trying to do their best, but they're solving the problem the wrong way for the wrong people. I watch well-meaning advocates raising funds to get people across state lines for abortion care that is no longer available or soon won't be in half the states in our nation, including my own state of Arizona, where a total ban on abortion except to save the life of the pregnant person was enforced for a time while writing this book and continues to be battled in court. I am unsure of what the outcome will be by the time this book is published. Hopefully the tide is turning with the reelection of Democrat senator Mark Kelly and the election of Democrat governor Katie Hobbs in November 2022. Their elections give me hope that Arizonans will continue to elect new local leaders who will work with our communities to expand access to healthcare instead of taking it away. Meanwhile, this fundraising work to help Arizonans travel to get the care they need is meaningful and important. Yet throwing money at getting people out of state for abortions isn't a long-term solution. There are barriers we can't buy our way around. We can't fund people around no days off. We can't fund people into being safe to travel. We can't fund people into having suitable child caregivers. Thus, the poorest and most vulnerable people are once again the ones forced to stay pregnant. One young couple who were able to self-fund to fly out of state for emergency abortion care put it like this:

It was through the experience of being denied care in our state and then understanding how incredibly lucky we were to be able to surmount the various barriers to getting on a plane last minute, booking last minute hotels, paying thousands and thousands of dollars out of pocket for the care itself ... trying to put all the pieces together in the moment and right away. I mean, we were on that plane thinking, what do people do who don't have a mom to borrow money from? Who don't have IDs so they can fly? Who might speak English as a second language? ... [we were] going through all of the various privileges that were required for us to surmount this abortion ban that we didn't know existed until we were in the moment and desperately needed care.

Beyond *Roe*: From Reproductive Choice to Reproductive Justice

Roe gave the very minimal right to abortion care, but it did not actually provide meaningful access to abortion for everyone who needed it. What good is a right if it can't be exercised?

For fifty years, *Roe* worked for white, cisgender women with the means to get childcare, time off work, and so on, but it never truly helped the people who found themselves too remote, endangered, or poor to access care.

In moving beyond Roe to something better, we must center the most marginalized, impacted people and their communities in a way that helps and engages them.

The definition of insanity is doing things the same way and expecting different results. The mission now cannot be to reinstate *Roe*. Now is the time to embrace a new framework to talk about abortion and access to abortion care. We can't silo abortion care into its own arena, separate from all the other issues affecting people. When we talk about whether or not to bring children into this world, we need to talk about lack of childcare, unsafe housing and neighborhoods, food deserts, unreliable transportation, toxic environments, lack of insurance, and so on.

WE CAN'T SILO ABORTION CARE INTO ITS OWN ARENA, SEPARATE FROM ALL THE OTHER ISSUES AFFECTING PEOPLE.

These conditions are called social determinants of health: the economic and social conditions outside of an individual's control that cause differences in health status. When we think and speak out about how pregnancy and abortion care intersect with a person's social determinants of health, we expand the conversation from reproductive choice to reproductive justice. As activist Loretta Ross has written,

> "The ability of any woman to determine her own reproductive destiny is directly linked to the conditions in her community, and these conditions are not just a matter of individual choice and access. For example, a woman cannot make an individual decision about her body if she is part of a community whose human rights as a group are violated, such as

through environmental dangers or insufficient quality health care."

When we see issues through this lens, we acknowledge that some people don't have choice, because they and their communities are being oppressed. Reproductive oppressions—the regulation and exploitation of an individual's sexuality, labor, and procreative capacities as a strategy to control individuals and community—can include the following:

1. Forced pregnancy
2. Forced sterilization
3. Health neglect
4. Violence
5. Mass incarceration

Focusing on justice, oppressions, and community creates a new narrative and a new language that's emotional enough and that touches enough daily lives that people like my staff member who didn't know what *Roe* was will pay attention. It shifts the conversation from abstract rights to everyday justice.

The way forward is to see the human right to an abortion through the lens of reproductive justice.

The reproductive justice framework engages people in their everyday lives and centers the people who need help the most. But before we can embrace this new framework, we have to understand what went wrong with the old.

The Problem of Choice

The mainstream women's movement of the 1970s that brought us *Roe* was focused on the concerns of white, middle-class, cisgender women. It was framed as pro-choice because this type of woman had a choice: she could stay home with her children or not. She could access abortion care or not. Meanwhile, millions of people found themselves in situations without any choice at all. They had to work to survive, so staying home to raise children wasn't really ever a choice. Abortion care often wasn't a choice, either, because ever-growing restrictions and lack of resources put access out of reach.

> The right to bodily autonomy—whether to have an abortion or to have and raise a child in safe conditions—was never reality for many people, especially the poor and people of color.

The scholar Marlene Fried breaks down why this narrow focus on "choice" was destined to fail:

1. Choice sets up a simple for-against divide. Reproductive issues are more complex, involving multiple human rights issues.
2. Choice is about the right not to have a child, but it ignores eugenics, population control, and the right to parent in safe communities. That is, many people are fighting for the right to *have* and safely raise children.
3. Choice was framed as antigovernment ("keep the government out of our wombs!") in order to appeal to conservatives. Justice demands the involvement of the government.

4. Choice didn't solve the problems of capitalism. If you didn't have money, you really didn't have a choice in America's privatized medical system.

5. Choice is about individuals. It ignores community and social barriers that prevent people from accessing their rights.

6. Choice is about people who have privilege, not the marginalized or oppressed.

7. Choice is not a powerful moral argument in the face of "life."

8. Choice is not a compelling enough vision to sustain an activist, grassroots movement.

In fact, the rhetoric of choice was not even motivating enough for the mainstream movement. The majority of pro-choice women remained on the sidelines while *Roe* was eroded by 1,381 restrictions. Katha Pollitt, the author of *Pro,* called "the millions of pro-choice Americans who are so far uninvolved (and still complacent)" the "muddled middle." These are people who vaguely believe in the abstract right to abortion but who aren't motivated to get out on the streets or into the voting booth to support that belief. Many of these people feel that while abortion is an okay choice for others, they wouldn't have an abortion themselves, and so their motivation to stand up and act is low. I believe that many of these people know deep down that they don't need to stand up for abortion rights for others because when it comes down to their own choice, they have the means and the privilege to access care despite government interference. History tells us that when the state regulates and criminalizes anything, including reproduction, white, well-off, cisgender women aren't going to be the ones who end up in prison.

The Birth of a Movement: Reproductive Justice

While mainstream feminist groups continued to focus on choice, groups like the National Black Feminist Organization, the Third World Women's Alliance, and the Committee for Abortion Rights and Against Sterilization Abuse were focusing on wider issues. They tried to talk about the Hyde Amendment (the banning of federal funds for abortion care), forced sterilization, unsafe neighborhoods, and how their struggles intersected with human rights struggles around the world, but their interests were treated as secondary at best.

In 1994, the term *reproductive justice* was coined by a group of American Black women in Chicago who founded Women of African Descent for Reproductive Justice. They defined reproductive justice as follows:

> The right to have children.
> The right not to have children.
> The right to nurture the children we have in a safe and healthy environment.

While the first point and second points were important, the third was revolutionary. It shined a light on people's actual lives and how those lives could be reenvisioned within the framework of a value-led society. It was an urgent call to directly link human rights and reproductive rights.

Three years later, in 1997, SisterSong was founded. This collective led by sixteen separate POC-headed organizations came together to support reproductive health for women of color. It included Native American, African American, Latine, and Asian American leadership. Loretta Ross, a cofounder of SisterSong, explained the need for the new movement: "Reducing women's lives down to just whether or not choice is available we felt was inadequate … choice and abortion … that's all they wanted to talk about."

Reproductive justice activists had more on their minds. Reproductive justice is an intersectional theory. It focuses on how the ability to determine one's own reproductive destiny is linked directly to the conditions of one's community. These conditions are not a matter of individual choice and access. They are not about a person's demand for privacy or bodily autonomy. Instead, reproductive justice focuses on the social forces that are outside of a person's individual control. It takes the blame and responsibility off the individual person and puts it squarely where it belongs: on society and its values.

Reproductive Justice on the Ground

I was born, raised, and trained in Los Angeles, California. I received my doctor of medicine degree from UCLA through a program with Charles R. Drew University, the only historically Black college west of the Mississippi. Charles Drew was founded as a response to the Watts Rebellion in Los Angeles in 1965, in which racial violence due to decades of oppression exploded over six days, causing $40 million in property damage and thirty-four deaths, mostly the "justifiable homicides" of Black people by the police and National Guard.

While in medical school and residency, I planned to stay in Los Angeles to serve the underserved predominantly Black and Latine population that was still experiencing the same inequities that had spurred the Rebellion almost four decades earlier. When I eventually left Los Angeles for Phoenix in 2009, that mission and vision for my life continued. In 2013, I founded Desert

DESERT STAR EXISTS TO PROMOTE THE HEALTH AND WELL-BEING OF OUR PATIENTS AND COMMUNITY.

Star Family Planning Clinic in Phoenix, Arizona, to combat the stigma that surrounds reproductive healthcare while bringing services to a medically underserved and ethnically diverse community. Desert Star exists to promote the health and well-being of our patients and community by providing just, dignified, and exceptional patient-centered care steeped in the philosophy of reproductive justice:

> Desert Star envisions a world where womb-bearing people can access the full range of reproductive health care regardless of circumstance or zip code. We are a steadfast resource for comprehensive family planning and sexual health care, a provider of long-term birth control to uninsured people, a safe and welcoming space for non-English speaking people, queer, transgender, gender nonconforming, and nonbinary people, and a hub for abortion training.

People often ask me what made me open an abortion clinic in a hostile state like Arizona. Now with the fall of *Roe*, they ask why I stay. The answer is simple. My strong sense of social justice leads me to serve the underserved, and I do this by executing on my vision of how the most marginalized people accessing abortion care deserve to feel and be treated. As a Black woman, there are many moments in my life when I have to decide to step up or accept the status quo. When I stepped up, I knew that I was finally saying yes to my community and my calling. I will not abandon either of those now.

My practice is my ministry. It is a combination of my spirituality and deep regard for justice.

In 2017, I founded Desert Star Institute for Family Planning, a nonprofit to complement the clinic's services. We've expanded from a destination for justice-centered abortion training to a resource for supplying long-term contraceptives to uninsured people, reproductive health education, and engagement and activism within marginalized communities. To date, close to one hundred people from nineteen states and three regions of Canada have trained with me at Desert Star Institute. The organization has evolved into a public-facing reproductive justice organization whose mission is to create equitable access to reproductive healthcare for womb-bearing people while centering Black, Indigenous, and other people of color. We form intentional partnerships and programming to build community and center marginalized voices.

The Day-to-Day of Reproductive Justice

By centering my work around equitable access to healthcare for marginalized people, I understand that I am called to do more than "be a doctor." There are three main frameworks to address reproductive oppression. In my clinic, my nonprofit, and my life, I am privileged to be able to work on all three:

> Reproductive health (service delivery): How will we deliver the care people need?
> Reproductive rights (legal advocacy): How will we keep care legal and accessible?
> Reproductive justice (organizing): How can we address social issues as they intersect with reproductive health?

Service delivery is what we do every day. At Desert Star, our team is small but mighty. We are never just doing procedures or treating conditions. We honor that there is an entire human being in front of us whom we need to see and acknowledge. We take the time to understand and to help that person understand how whatever they've come to us for is intersecting with the rest of their life.

Looking at a patient's situation through the lens of reproductive justice can be as simple as being compassionate around lateness to appointments due to unreliable transportation, unpredictable childcare, or lack of flexibility at jobs. When clinics and doctors' offices uphold strict fifteen-minutes-late-and-you're-out or no-children-in-waiting-room policies, we hurt the people who need care the most. Acknowledging that these rules are often beyond an individual doctor's control, it is a system-wide culture that fails to center the patients who are trying to receive care. I also understand that not all my patients have access to state-issued IDs, a problem in most medical settings. All these "minor" problems are social determinants of health: social issues intersecting with healthcare issues. Transportation, childcare, and access to service are all problems reproductive justice addresses.

On a deeper level, reproductive justice means that when we deliver care, patients get a say in everything we do. They get to ask questions and engage in a dialogue. As a gynecologist, I always hold top of mind the history of physician J. Marion Sims and his barbaric experimentation on enslaved women who could not consent. I am constantly aware of the current, ongoing racism that believes Black bodies do not experience pain in the way that white bodies do. I understand Black women's lived experiences of racist tropes like being considered hypersexual "Jezebels" and how those attitudes extend to the exam room. I understand that most procedures I do will cause pain and discomfort, so before I act, I explain. I also take the time to make things less painful when possible. For example, I've picked up techniques that make IUD insertion less painful. Often, patients who have had insertions before tell me "Oh my God, this was so much better."

Paying attention and caring about pain is part of decolonizing my practice. It's interesting to me that I often see pain reduction discussed in Black female gynecologist forums and rarely elsewhere. I believe we as Black physicians are more in tune with this issue because before we became doctors, we experienced the same kinds of racist treatment that our patients do now. I clearly remember being sixteen and being told by the practitioner performing my first ever speculum examination, "Relax, it's just like sex." Even then

I BELIEVE WE AS BLACK PHYSICIANS ARE MORE IN TUNE WITH THIS ISSUE [OF PAIN REDUCTION] BECAUSE BEFORE WE BECAME DOCTORS, WE EXPERIENCED THE SAME KINDS OF RACIST TREATMENT THAT OUR PATIENTS DO NOW.

I thought, *Well, it's not. And would you have said that to a sixteen-year-old white girl?* Now, even though we're physicians, we continue to encounter racism within healthcare settings, especially before our white colleagues know we're doctors.

When it comes to abortion, the procedure itself usually does not require much physical healing. A typical first-trimester abortion takes about five minutes and is minimally invasive. My patients sometimes request first-trimester abortions without sedation because they need to get back to work that same night. But there is emotional and spiritual pain that we take the time to acknowledge and discuss. I consider abortion care an act of love. We acknowledge that people have to go through deep healing because of the harmful religious and social rhetoric surrounding them. This is emotional and spiritual warfare that people are fighting. They often think they're fighting against themselves and don't realize they're fighting against a powerful and organized antiabortion movement that doesn't care about their well-being despite protestations to the contrary. They are fighting against a racist and patriarchal society that not only doesn't help them but actively harms them in all sorts of insidious ways that they might not be aware of. And, of course, they're fighting against a government that believes it has an interest in their pregnancy, leading to potential policing and punishment, particularly if they're members of already overpoliced communities. Everything we do and say acknowledges these realities. We join them in these fights, linking medical care and social justice in individual patient care and in our broader work outside the exam room doors.

Linking Advocacy, Activism, and Healthcare

Another way we bring social justice to healthcare is during doctor training. Traditional medical education is problem and system based. Approaching the care of a patient from a reproductive justice standpoint means that I teach my trainees that they're not just treating a specific medical condition. They must look at the person's entire reality and the conditions of their life that contribute to the problem.

> To really make a patient's life better, doctors need to be addressing and advocating to improve the conditions that created the situation to begin with.

As it relates to abortion care, there can be many issues at play. Maybe the person already has children who they are having trouble feeding, clothing, and housing, and they don't want to add to that familial burden. We need to address whether they have a living wage, health insurance, childcare, and so on. All those issues affect how they decide whether or not to add to their family in that moment with that particular pregnancy. In other words, we make social determinants of health an integral part of reproductive healthcare.

> When doctors center their work around equitable access to healthcare for marginalized people, then they understand that being a physician means they are called to do more than just "be a doctor."

When I train medical students and residents, I am actively culti-vating advocates for reproductive health and justice in the communi-ties they serve. I'm not just giving hands-on skills to future doctors. I believe their patients and their communities are going to be better for that. As Dr. Becca Simon, a doctor with whom I have a peer and trainee relationship, explains, "When I was in training, I realized how critical abortion care is to the health of a community … Doing this work has transformed me. I wish people knew that abortion providers are people who really care about the communities they live in … Abortions are essential healthcare. When we restrict bodily autonomy, it can change the course of a pregnant person's life."

LGBTQ+ and Reproductive Justice

Another way we bring reproductive justice into the clinic is by actively providing meaningful access and support to LGBTQ+ reproductive healthcare. In my clinic, I understand that everyone has some type of oppression that they're facing. I am intersectional, always looking to find where oppressions overlap so we can work together toward a common goal.

One example of this is how the reproductive health of trans people is currently playing out in the abortion debate. There are many cisgender women who don't want to include trans men in the discussion of abortion care. They believe that we are erasing women by saying "pregnant people" instead of "women." Instead of seeing things from this position of opposition, we need to understand that we can walk and chew gum at the same time. We can include everyone within an intersectional framework. We can respect and uphold one group's rights without canceling another's. We have to create that intersectional narrative and push people until they understand, because separating and acting narrowly has never succeeded. Bringing more people under the umbrella only helps us all.

Other Modalities of Care

Focusing on reproductive justice also invites midwives, doulas, and community health workers into the reproductive healthcare conversation. For centuries, the medical community has actively worked against these types of practitioners. The history of opposition to abortion in America began with male medical doctors actively wanting to prohibit these mostly female, "nonprofessional" caregivers from infringing on what they perceived as their turf. Reproductive justice brings these essential care providers back into the conversation.

> When we focus on communities, we focus on raising up the traditional wisdom that resides within communities.

This helps everyone. One 2016 study in the journal *Birth* showed that women who received doula support had a 22 percent lower chance of preterm and cesarean births. Michelle Ivette Ponce, cofounder of Arizona Birthworkers of Color, explains what care that is focused on reproductive justice looks like in her group's work:

> Birthworkers show up when a person is going to have a baby. We have birth doulas that help with birth and abortion doulas who support a family or person when they're having an abortion. We're offering families a way to empower themselves beyond expecting the government and our politicians to help us. Birth workers are in a beautiful space to be able to do that. They get to go into people's homes and really understand what's going on. The barriers to wellness are many: criminalization, white supremacy, extreme religion, capitalism. There's a lot of shame. We hide our stories. There's a history of silence in our families and in our communities. There's a lot of miseducation about sex, about maternal health, about what to do when you're pregnant. We have the power and the information to overcome those barriers. Birth workers are trained to inform our clients, sharing factual and research-based information. We can help find community resources like food banks or low-cost childcare. While we also work on changing policy and legislation, we know that sometimes what we have best is each other. We are here for each other. We can actually make a difference.

As abortion care becomes increasingly criminalized for both practitioners and those seeking care, the importance of practitioners who can operate outside the highly regulated, highly policed healthcare system grows. We already know that people of color will be disproportionately targeted under criminalization policies. Thus, in addition to physicians and publicly facing groups like Arizona Birthworkers of Color, who work within the law, there is also a growing movement of "below the grass roots" providers who exist in "the underground: a small network of community providers who connect with abortion seekers by word of mouth … Its ranks include midwives, herbalists, doulas, and educators. When necessary, they are often willing to work around the law." As we see abortion bans grow, these groups grounded in reproductive justice principles will grow as well.

> WE NEED TO UNDERSTAND THAT WE CAN WALK AND CHEW GUM AT THE SAME TIME. WE CAN INCLUDE EVERYONE WITHIN AN INTERSECTIONAL FRAMEWORK.

Reproductive Justice and Pregnancy as a Path to Criminality

When we make abortion illegal, we turn pregnant people, their physicians, birth workers, and now even friends and family into criminals. We know that marginalized people are already criminalized for unjust reasons, including being poor. In addition, so-called justice is not handed out equally among all people. There's no reason to expect any of this to be different as ever-more-stringent abortion laws are enforced. This will not only affect people who seek abortions. Vulnerable people will be overinvestigated for their miscarriages and for losing their babies. Their doctors, midwives, and doulas, especially if they're also from marginalized groups, will end up in prison for providing miscarriage and postbirth care.

Garin Marschall, cofounder of Patient Forward and RHAvote (Reproductive Health Act Vote), points out that "we know that when the state has an interest in something, it protects that interest with policing power, violence, and punishment. Abortion bans invite this power into our lives." Marschall asks, "Why is our society's reaction to problems to criminalize, surveil, and then punish? We need to move away from that as a response to social issues, especially abortion. There are other options that are more effective, better for our communities, and better for our well-being that we should be embracing and pursuing."

Reproductive justice offers these options. Reproductive justice is not about policing whether an abortion should occur. It instead asks if a birth should occur. Does this specific person, in this specific situation, have the ability to raise this specific child? The answer depends on focusing on the broader life and situation of everyone involved. Can we help people find health-care, childcare, a living wage? If they're bringing a disabled child into the world, will we support them in raising that child? Can this particular hospital provide for this particular medically fragile child? Or are we too far from the advanced technology and skilled practitioner care this particular child will need? When these are the questions, then the answers become clear: we need universal healthcare, subsidized childcare, housing equity, better physician training, increased funding for social safety nets, and so on.

> **ANTIABORTION FORCES CLAIM THEY'RE PRO-LIFE. REPRODUCTIVE JUSTICE EXPOSES THAT THEY'RE ONLY PRO-BIRTH.**

The Future of Reproductive Justice

Antiabortion forces claim they're pro-life. Reproductive justice exposes that they're only pro-birth. When we include the right to raise children in safe communities in our conversations, we shift the focus away from birth versus abortion and toward the actual lives of parents and children, taking the moral high ground from the other side. As pointed out by SisterSong, reproductive justice concerns "the way that the state and others refuse to support us with quality services and resources, but at the same time interferes in our lives and decisions." Reproductive justice understands that "reproductive oppression is a means of selectively controlling the destiny of entire communities through the bodies of women and individuals, a newer and more subtle form of negative eugenics."

While reproductive justice is a people of color–led movement, there is room for everyone to join this fight. Loretta Ross, speaking for SisterSong, explains how focusing on the most impacted people helps everyone:

> The U.S. system of white supremacy facilitates reproductive oppression ... for white women as well because their individual decisions are directly tied to their communities—in particular, racist fears triggered by the decreasing percentage of white children born in the United States. Many of the restrictions on abortion, contraception [and so on] ... are directly related to an unsubtle campaign of positive eugenics to force heterosexual white women to have more babies.... We must end the separation of abortion rights from other social justice, reproductive rights and human rights issues because it is difficult—if not impossible—to

mobilize communities in defense of abortion rights if abortion is taken out of the context of empowering women, creating healthier families, and promoting sustainable communities.

We can all be in this together if we understand that our future is connected: white people, people of color, LGBTQ+ people, disabled people, adoption rights advocates, physicians, midwives, doulas, community health workers, rural residents, urban residents, red states, blue states, and so on. Until we join together, we'll keep failing. We can't allow this moment to pass us by. We don't live in a society in which every child born is loved and has the resources to grow and thrive. We can change this, but only if we change the conversation. People aren't making the decision to have an abortion in a vacuum but within the context of their lives. We need to start seeing it that way, talking about it that way, and creating solutions that account for people's whole lives. Reproductive justice shows us the way.

TALKING ABOUT REPRODUCTIVE JUSTICE

Myth: *Roe* **gave us the right to abortion.**

Reality: "I agree with law professor Dr. Khiara Bridges who says *Roe* gave us the right to buy an abortion if you can find one and can afford it."

Myth: Reproductive healthcare ends when babies are born.

Reality: "If the state is going to force me to give birth in a historically and systemically racist, ablest, homophobic, paternalist, and economically unjust society, I'm going to need a lot of help with that."

Myth: Helping women in states where abortion is banned looks like helping them travel across state lines.

Reality: "I couldn't possibly leave my kids and my job while I traveled out of state for an abortion. I'm so thankful for the grassroots, community-based support that reached me where I am."

Myth: It's not the state's job to support parents who can't support themselves.

Reality: "The state causes problems by passing unjust laws and enforcing them inequitably with violence, incarceration, and coercion. Either they need to get out of my reproductive life, or they need to support mothers and children. They can't have it both ways."

Myth: Doctors can be "just doctors."

Reality: "I experienced so many barriers trying to undergo care in a traditional healthcare setting, I almost gave up. Being seen by a physician steeped in my realities not only made a huge difference in my care, but it made me become an activist myself."

Myth: Reproductive justice fights only for poor people and people of color.

Reality: "The fight for racial justice, economic justice, disability justice, LGBTQ+ justice, women's justice, and so on are all connected. Bringing these fights together under one roof makes us all stronger. When we win for the most vulnerable among us, everyone wins."

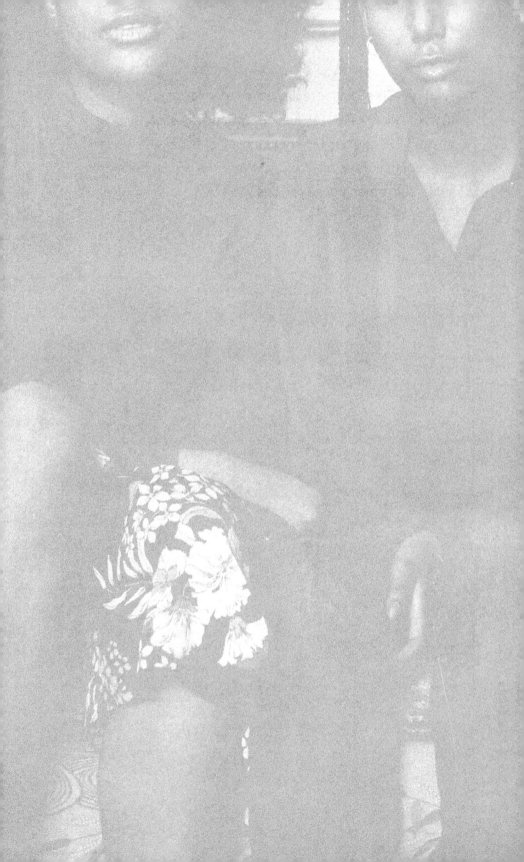

CHAPTER SEVEN

REAL HARM

Antiabortion Tactics and How to Fight Them

"Many states, like California, are legalizing infanticide."

I came across this remarkable "fact" in a comment on a friend's Facebook post. Often, I leave this sort of thing be. It's just not worth the trouble. But this was a long thread with almost seventy comments, so I knew there were a lot of people reading this nonsense.

I replied "Stop it," to which the commenter supplied a link to an article from a right-wing, antiabortion "news" outlet with the headline "California Bill Would Allow Killing Babies in Infanticide Up to 28 Days After Birth." It was accompanied by a picture of a sleeping infant.

As ridiculous as it was, I wasn't surprised to see this headline or picture. Fearmongering over nonexistent infanticide wasn't isolated to this outlet, which mediabiasfactcheck.com calls a "questionable source" due to "the use of poor sources, promotion of pseudoscience, and numerous failed fact-checks." I had already gotten a call from a legitimate AP reporter fact-checking the story that was spreading quickly across the internet. Reuters reported a Twitter post of a similar article with over six thousand reactions, including "A tsunami of evil is sweeping the West. I can't even begin to comprehend the depths of this depravity" and "I can't wrap my head around this … Is this for real or some sick joke or fake news?"

It was fake news. There was a California bill, AB2223, intended to ensure that people who experience miscarriages, still births, and perinatal deaths of their babies due to pregnancy complications weren't prosecuted as criminals. The disinformation over infanticide arose around language in the draft bill that prohibited civil or criminal prosecution for "perinatal death due to a pregnancy-related cause." The dictionary definition of *perinatal* is the period "just before, during, or within days or weeks of birth." This allowed pro-life extremists to pounce. They took the word out of context to make the wild claim that parents could murder their month-old babies, which of course was never the case. As the bill's sponsor, Buffy Wicks, explained on Twitter, "Let me be clear: #AB2223 doesn't prevent the state from keeping children safe. This isn't a bill about infanticide. This is about protecting Californians who suffer pregnancy loss from being unjustly investigated, prosecuted, or incarcerated. Full stop." This bill existed because pregnant people—usually marginalized people—were ending up in prison because of heartbreaking medical tragedies.

To end the hysteria, lawmakers reworded the final bill to make absolutely clear that it concerned only "perinatal death due to causes that occurred in utero." This, of course, had the exact same meaning as the original phrase "due to a pregnancy-related cause" but made doubly explicit what was already stated in the bill for people who took the time to carefully read it: infanticide is illegal.

Careful isn't what fake news is about. It's about sensationalism and riling up people's emotions. To understand why this bill existed and why the language *perinatal* was included, you have to go deep. But who is going to read assembly bills and explore the reasons behind them? Here is the real issue: not all pregnancies end in live birth, and not all babies survive.

- Miscarriage: 15–20 percent of pregnancies end in miscarriage—pregnancy loss before the twentieth week.

- Stillbirth: 1 in 160 births end in stillbirth, the loss of a pregnancy after the twentieth week—24,000 babies a year.

- Perinatal: another 4 in 1,000 babies die in the first twenty-eight days of life, usually due to premature birth, low birthweight, and birth defects.

As antiabortion laws increase, every one of these losses becomes a potential criminal event. The National Advocates for Pregnant Women reports that "pregnancy criminalization has more than tripled across the country in recent years to include more than 1,300 cases from 2006 through 2020 ... And from the 1973 *Roe v. Wade* ruling through 2020, NAPW has documented more than 1,700 cases

ALL THIS LEADS TO PREGNANT PEOPLE ... GETTING CAUGHT UP IN THE CRIMINAL JUSTICE SYSTEM FOR THE LOSS OF THEIR PREGNANCIES OR THE DEATH OF THEIR BABIES.

of arrests, prosecutions, detentions, or forced medical interventions carried out against pregnant people." The CDC reports that stillbirths are more common in Black pregnant people and those from low socio-economic communities. In addition, non-Hispanic Black people have 2.3 times the infant mortality rate as non-Hispanic whites.

All this leads to pregnant people, especially Black people and other marginalized groups, facing the growing possibility of getting caught up in the criminal justice system for the loss of their pregnancies or the death of their babies soon after. Two high-profile cases in California where women were sent to prison for stillbirths focused attention on the issue. The fear of an unequally applied justice system leads vulnerable people who need medical care the most not to seek it due to fear of prosecution and persecution. So while there was no valid reason for anyone to worry about a "depraved," imaginary free-for-all of unpunished, evil Californian infanticides, there was every reason to worry about the criminalization of pregnancy loss that this bill was trying to address.

This is why the bill was proposed and why California AB2223 was signed into law by the governor September 27, 2022.

It was impossible for me to get all that into a Facebook comment thread, so even though the bill succeeded, the harm of the lies swirling around it continues to grow. This was the intention. None of this was ever about whether infanticide was actually happening. It was about creating an emotional response. If antiabortion extremists can get somebody to believe that babies who have already been born are being killed, then abortion supporters are depraved people, the same people who are killing babies in utero. These activists wanted people to think, *See, if we allow abortions to happen, then they're just going down the slippery slope to kill actual babies who have been born.* The nonexistent "issue" of infanticide succeeds in painting proabortion supporters as depraved, sick, evil, and less than human.

Disinformation is a game that's being played to affect how people think about abortions, the people who provide them, and the people who have them.

Extremists purposefully use disinformation to dehumanize abortion supporters, creating space for violence, injustice, and division. It works. They were able to enrage and mobilize an army of people like the one who posted the link to the lie, someone who surely never took the time to figure out what they were supporting and why.

But antiabortion fervor is not the only harm. The lies also succeed in distracting people from the very real problems of skyrocketing miscarriage, stillbirth, infant mortality, and the criminalization of pregnancy, especially in Black and other marginalized communities. These problems are hard to solve. They're complex. They require that we all come together to see one another as partners in the struggle to improve conditions for everyone. As long as the lies proliferate, none of that will happen. Well-meaning but misinformed people will continue to fight on the internet and in other arenas over nonsense while real tragedies are happening to real people.

This chapter will explore some of the most damaging fake news, outright lies, clever deceptions, and other tactics of antiabortion extremists that create real harm for real individuals and communities. Knowing what their strategies are, who supports them, and who spreads them allows us to combat them. Understanding the danger is a first step in making the world a better, safer place for pregnant people and their families.

The Danger: Fake News

The harm: Proabortion forces are demonized; real issues are ignored; clickbait and other forms of sensationalism are rewarded with dollars. **The fix:** Learn the real facts; engage when constructive; resist the emotional clickbait.

It would take a whole book to address all the fake news invented by antiabortion extremists. A few examples of the false narratives that are being spread: abortion is dangerous to women, you can "reverse" a medical abortion, abortion clinics are unsafe, abortions are being performed "seconds" before birth, abortion leads to depression and suicide, abortion causes cancer, a six-week-old fetus can feel pain, abortion doctors rake in huge profits, abortion is Black genocide, and so on.

When you come across these sorts of stories, it doesn't always make sense to engage. You'll never change the mind of a person who has been convinced, and confrontation often drives these sorts of people deeper into their beliefs. Fact-checking is meaningless to people who believe that they "know" the truth. However, if you're in a public forum, like social media, it can help to engage and help others who are reading to understand that the narratives are false. It's important to choose your battles. Limit your engagement to posts with a lot of comments or likes that indicate others are lurking who can take the message in.

> Being the countervoice that calls out lies educates the silent people watching who can be reached.

To protect yourself from becoming influenced by the lies, it's important to understand that if you're reading something that's making you feel emotional, especially as it relates to abortion, take an extra step to check the validity. Extremists are so successful in their messaging because their "facts" are designed to be heartbreaking. The stories and lies they tell have been carefully crafted to evoke an emotional response. They've done a great deal of research into understanding human nature, and so they understand that emotions override the logical mind. Sensationalism manipulates people, and it's very powerful. The length that the antiabortion movement has gone to analyze how people think, then to use that to further their own agendas and keep particular people in power, is honestly disgusting. The people who follow these groups don't realize that a level of brainwashing has occurred. They believe that they're having independent thought on a matter when they're literally regurgitating talking points found in any right-wing publication.

If you are somebody who cares about someone who has fallen down a rabbit hole of conspiracy beliefs, presenting them with information that counters their belief only makes them more entrenched. The only way that impacted people change their minds is if something actually happens to them or someone they care deeply about. And even then, it often doesn't change their thinking. All we can do is arm ourselves with accurate information to reach the people on the fence, who may not have formed opinions on the issue one way or the other.

There is a vacuum of people who actually believe in a person's ability to exercise bodily autonomy and choose abortion. Most abortion supporters are ambivalent and don't have much to say. People feel that it's not their business whether somebody has an abortion or not. They think, *People should be able to do what they want, so why should I say anything about it?* That void is filled with a very eager minority of people who have a lot to say that is blatantly false.

We are in a moment right now when it's important for people in the majority to make their voices heard. The way to have an intelligent conversation about these things is to participate. Actively go out and seek the correct information. When you do engage, keep it simple. Don't answer emotion with emotion. Emphasize that abortion is basic healthcare, and it should be affordable. It's the everyday that's really a tragedy—that people can't access the care they need. People shouldn't have to provide tragedy porn to convince others that the abortion they're seeking is valid.

Unfortunately, there's an idea that we have to counter sensational lies with sensational truths. Instead, the message should be that abortion care is healthcare.

I have a friend who spends a great deal of time very successfully engaging with people who aren't completely to the extreme side but who lean that way—people who abstractly believe abortions shouldn't happen. On a Facebook thread, she had an interaction with someone who she knew personally who posted that she thought abortion should be illegal. My friend wrote, *If abortion is illegal, then the natural consequence of someone having one is prison. I had an abortion. Do you believe that I belong in prison?* They kept going back and forth, and my friend kept asking, *Do you believe that I should be in prison?* Finally, their friend admitted that seemed extreme. My friend wrote, *Then you don't want abortion to be illegal.* We live in a country that incarcerates the most people in the world. Once you make something illegal, more people end up in prison. When this sort of conversation happens between two people of color, the unstated becomes clear: *we end up in prison.* That sort of logical, calm engagement can shift people's mindset. The more voices we have, the more minds that can be changed.

The Danger: Fake Clinics

The harm: Harmful medical advice, siphoning of tax dollars meant to help women and children, disappearance of real clinics

The fix: Report fake clinics to databases and on social media; inform your friends, family, and community; contact your local lawmakers to demand regulation and public defunding of fake clinics; take direct action against fake clinics in your community; find your real clinic and support it.

I recently had a patient come to my clinic with an ultrasound that was so badly done, we had to repeat the procedure. I asked her where she'd gotten it, but I already knew—at a fake health clinic. These so-called crisis pregnancy centers are purposefully designed to look like licensed medical facilities, but they aren't. They are usually staffed with volunteers or employees who almost always lack sufficient medical training. They have one purpose: to stop people from getting abortions. As www. exposefakeclinics.com explains, "Fake clinics do NOT provide comprehensive reproductive health care—or much of any 'health care' at all! Instead, they use phony ads to trick pregnant people into making an appointment, promising 'free ultrasounds' or 'pregnancy support.' Once inside, people are lied to, shamed, and pressured about their reproductive health decisions, often delaying their procedure, or pushing them past the deadline for a legal abortion altogether." By the time patients get to me, they're often distressed and grossly misinformed.

Exposefakeclinics.com quotes an antiabortion activist who explains how it works:

> Women seeking abortions, women that are pregnant, that are vulnerable, they are going into Google, and they are typing 'pregnancy symptoms.' There's a way in Google where you can basically set that search to your website ... We want to look professional ... business-like. And, yeah, we do kind of want to look medical. The best client you ever get is one that thinks they're walking into an abortion clinic.
>
> **—Abby Johnson,** antichoice activist
> at a fake clinic training

In other words, these clinics are designed to deceive. The Gutt-macher Institute documents some of the most common forms of disinformation given to people lured inside in search of accurate medical care:

- Disinformation that abortion increases breast cancer, infertility, and mental health issues

- Dishonest delaying tactics meant to put abortion out of reach, either, because of time-limit laws or the increased costs that later abortions incur

- Inaccurate information about contraception in order to promote abstinence

Bad medical advice is rampant in these centers to promote their singular goal of convincing people to stay pregnant. I see patients who have been misinformed over how far along their pregnancy is or patients who have been encouraged to continue dangerous ectopic pregnancies that can never result in live birth and can kill the pregnant person. The Women's Law Project found that in Pennsylvania, "32.0% of CPCs [crisis pregnancy centers] provide, refer for, or promote 'abortion pill reversal' (APR). APR is the unrecognized practice of injecting or prescribing high-dose progesterone for pregnant people who have taken the first medicine in the two-step protocol for medication abortion in an attempt to stop ('reverse') the abortion. The American College of Obstetricians and Gynecologists calls APR 'unethical' and 'not based on science.' This rogue practice has been called 'unproven and experimental' in *The New England Journal of Medicine* because neither the safety nor effectiveness of APR has been proven in clinical trials." Because these fake clinics often operate in minority communities, this is an example of the continuation of racist medical experimentation on marginalized people.

There are three thousand fake clinics in America, and the number is growing. Fake clinics outnumber real abortion providers by an average of three to one, and in some states as much as nine to one.

These "pregnancy crisis centers" or "pregnancy resource centers" are often set up next to real medical clinics to purposely cause confusion. They often operate in low-income or minority communities, targeting those least likely to see through their tactics. Because they often aren't licensed health facilities, they don't have to follow the rules of real clinics, which must uphold medical board standards. In other words, they can mislead or omit information to serve their hidden agenda. In addition, they don't have to follow HIPAA privacy laws because those only apply to real medical facilities, an increasingly dangerous situation as pregnancy becomes increasingly criminalized.

FAKE CLINICS OUTNUMBER REAL ABORTION PROVIDERS BY AN AVERAGE OF THREE TO ONE, AND IN SOME STATES AS MUCH AS NINE TO ONE.

These clinics are amazingly often supported by tax dollars. Take a moment to think about that: your money is being spent to deliberately mislead people to carry out an antiabortion agenda. The Associated Press reports that in 2022 "nearly $89 million has been allocated to such centers across about a dozen states this fiscal year. A decade ago, the annual funding for the programs hovered around $17 million in about eight states." Most alarming, at least ten states take these millions of dollars in block grant money that was specifically intended to go directly to needy families in the form of welfare or TANF (Temporary Assistance for Needy Families).

Contrast this with the situation of real reproductive healthcare medical clinics. Three out of five people have abortion care at an independent clinic, yet 133 independent abortion clinics have been forced to close since 2017 due to excessive regulation, lack of funds, or other government interference. Fourteen states are without a single abortion-providing clinic. Independent clinics are closing at an alarming rate. No state has been without at least one clinic since ACN started tracking abortion clinics in 2012. As the Abortion Care Network points out, independent providers are "the most vulnerable to anti-abortion attacks and legislation intended to close clinic doors or push abortion out of reach." Real clinics provide more than abortions. They are often a community's best access to all reproductive healthcare, including contraception, preventive healthcare, prenatal care, OB-GYN care, and other important services. When they disappear, people aren't just losing access to abortion care but to healthcare. When these clinics are gone, we know that they rarely come back.

IN EXCHANGE FOR SOME EXTRA SEATS IN A STADIUM ... ARIZONA HAS ALLOWED ... LAWMAKERS TO PROHIBIT FOR DECADES THE TEACHING OF ABORTION IN ONE OF ITS MAJOR PUBLIC UNIVERSITIES.

Desert Star, my clinic, is a good example of the challenges real independent clinics face. With every onerous regulation passed, my clinic becomes more expensive to operate. We aren't heavily resourced. We're operating on margins that don't allow us to withstand even small increases in overhead due to growing regulation, inflation, or increased wages for staff in tight labor markets. And yet we exist without public funds to serve the community, providing real medical services that save lives. I am committed to keeping my doors open to serve my community, but statistics show I'm fighting an uphill battle.

Exposing the harm of fake clinics takes work. If you see a fake clinic, report it to exposefakeclinics.com. Share it on social media at #badfaithmedicine or #exposefakeclinics. Educate your friends, family, and community. Contact your local lawmakers to demand regulation of fake clinics. While you're at it, demand defunding of fake clinics if public funding exists in your state. If you're willing to go further, reproductive justice groups like Reproaction have detailed information on how to take direct action against fake clinics in your area.

Then find your real independent clinic and support it. You can give money or volunteer. Even if you have no medical skills, independent clinics need people to do nonmedical tasks that require minimal training, like helping patients fill out intake forms or perform pregnancy tests. Other proactive ways to support your local clinic are detailed in chapter 9.

The Danger: Control of Healthcare Access and Medical Training by Antiabortion Forces

The harm: Lack of trained doctors, denial of essential healthcare.

The fix: Demand your institutions and politicians don't accept money with strings attached, be aware of religious institutions that won't perform basic healthcare, speak out against state laws that protect hospitals that deny lifesaving care, support hospitals and clinics that support abortion care.

I was at a fundraiser in Los Angeles where I met a man from Tucson, which is a liberal-leaning city in southern Arizona and home to the main campus of the University of Arizona. I shared with him the remarkable story of how in 1974, legislators were able to add a peculiar stipulation to a $5.5 million bond raising money to expand the university's football stadium. In exchange for the money, the university's medical school was prohibited from training students to do abortions. Amazingly, the state supreme court upheld the rider, and to this day, University of Arizona medical students have to get their abortion training from the local Planned Parenthood. In exchange for some extra seats in a stadium almost fifty years ago, Arizona has allowed some minor, local 1970s lawmakers to prohibit for decades the teaching of abortion in one of its major public universities.

The man I was speaking to, like most people outside the day-to-day battles with abortion opponents, was shocked. He had no idea. Why would he? Tucson is such a progressive city, so how could this happen there? And what does a football stadium have to do with abortion? Yet these sorts of funding-controlled arrangements are common in restricting abortion access and abortion training even in liberal bastions like Tucson.

> People need to be aware that there are very conservative forces that are actually running things in the background through funding decisions that restrict abortion access or training.

Religiously affiliated residency programs and hospitals are also big forces in restricting doctor training and abortion access. The ACLU reports that "one in six hospital beds in the U.S. is in a facility that complies with Catholic directives that prohibit a range of reproductive healthcare services, even when a woman's life or health is in jeopardy. In some states, more than 40 percent of all hospital beds are in a Catholic-run facility, leaving entire regions without any option for certain reproductive health care services." The control of so much of our health system by religious institutions often surprises people, and they are even more surprised when they realize that the trend is growing in blue states like Oregon, Washington, California, New York, and Connecticut. The horror stories of pregnant people being denied lifesaving care at these hospitals are harrowing and too many to go into here.

Religious institutions don't provide abortions or abortion training, and these groups certainly don't try to hide it. But most people don't think about who controls their hospital until they are denied training or care. Why would they? We care about rights, but we're also just living our lives, assuming that because most people support abortion, we'll be able to access care if we need it. But if a hospital is funded by an antiabortion religious group, that isn't the case.

The secondary scandal is the lack of training at these hospitals. One recent study published in the *American Journal of Obstetrics & Gynecology* found that nearly half of all Catholic and other religious hospitals fail to comply with required abortion and family planning training for obstetrics and gynecology residents. Only those who go above and beyond to seek abortion training get it.

But amazingly, it's not only religious hospitals that don't offer abortion-care training. It takes dedicated initiative from doctors, professors, and medical students to assure students get training. This training doesn't come without a cost. Trainees can slow down clinic flow and increase operational costs. I had a cost analysis done for my abortion training program at Desert Star. It costs $1,000 for a four-week rotation for a fourth-year medical student or resident to receive hands-on abortion training. Yet we need future abortion providers trained. With abortion bans being enforced in a third of the US as of the writing of this book, we need providers who may have taken a back seat in the past to stand up and teach in the places where abortion care is still available.

Stanford University researchers found that half of US medical schools included no formal abortion training or only a single lecture.

I see in my own experience the difference even a single person can make. I train students in Phoenix in my clinic and as a professor at the University of Arizona College of Medicine–Phoenix. I got my faculty appointment there, and in 2010 started giving the lecture on birth control for their reproductive health block. Before I came, there was a few minutes of birth control information thrown into a general gynecology lecture and nothing about abortion. Since then, I have slowly expanded what I teach. I now give three hours of lecture: an hour on hormonal birth control, an hour on nonhormonal birth control and emergency contraception, and an hour on diagnosis and management of unintended and abnormal pregnancy—that is, miscarriage and abortion. Because I advocated for it, those students went from having maybe ten to fifteen minutes of instruction on birth control in their second year of medical school to three hours of comprehensive instruction. That's unheard of. That's just not happening across the country. The average student is getting maybe thirty minutes over the entire first two years of basic medical science.

Medical students themselves can also play a role in changing the dire situation. The group Medical Students for Choice is a worthy force in helping to preserve abortion training and access. I am the faculty advisor for the Medical Students for Choice group at the University of Arizona College of Medicine–Phoenix, and I see the importance and strength of their community. However, the fact these groups even need to exist exposes the lack of access to training many medical students experience. We're in a dangerous time.

As soon as doctors can't perform abortions because they're illegal, then they can't train people.

We're in a moment when half the country is moving to ban abortion. Who are the abortion providers of the future if there's no training? Even if one doesn't "believe" in abortion, miscarriage management makes abortion care imperative. We are going to see impacts of this for generations. There won't be doctors able to meet the needs of people who need abortion care. When the pendulum swings back and abortion access is opened up again—as I believe it will be when the effects of the new laws become clear—the doctors won't be there.

TALKING ABOUT REAL HARM:

Myth: It's not worth engaging in abortion fights on social media.

Reality: "When I saw that post from my friend about abortion causing cancer, I was glad I added a calm, sane voice to the conversation. Maybe it won't matter, but maybe someone will read what I wrote and think twice."

Myth: It's illegal to pretend to be a healthcare clinic.

Reality: "The women at the pregnancy center wore white lab coats and gave me an ultrasound. It wasn't until later when they began calling me and telling me that I would die and end up in hell did I realize I'd been tricked—and that it was all perfectly legal."

Myth: Being in a blue state means I'll have abortion care when I need it.

Reality: "I was rushed to the nearest hospital when my water broke at eighteen weeks, before my fetus was viable. The Catholic hospital where I was taken gave me two Tylenol and sent me home. I only learned later that they knew that the baby couldn't possibly survive and that they hadn't helped me because of their religious beliefs. I didn't even know that could happen in America."

Myth: All doctors, especially ob-gyns, get training in contraception, miscarriage, and abortion care.

Reality: "It was almost impossible for me to get abortion training in my state. It's not offered at my medical school. It took me six months to find a provider willing to teach me, but then the clinic closed, the last in the state, and I was out of luck."

Myth: Tax dollars don't fund private, religious, anti-abortion organizations.

Reality: "I was shocked to learn that my state gives millions of dollars to 'abortion-alternative' organizations to promote their religious beliefs. We really ought to give that money to pregnant people or at least real care providers."

Myth: It's us against them, and anything goes in the fight.

Reality: "We need to find a way to come together to fight for people to get the healthcare they need. As long as we demonize one another, we'll never get to the real issues that can improve people's lives."

CHAPTER EIGHT

SUPPRESSION BY DESIGN

Voting and Politics

In the *Dobbs v. Jackson Women's Health Organization* opinion that overturned *Roe v. Wade*, Supreme Court Justice Samuel Alito wrote, "The permissibility of abortion, and the limitations upon it, are to be resolved like most important questions in our democracy: by citizens trying to persuade one another and then voting." Thirty-nine days later, on August 2, 2022, citizens in Kansas delivered a landslide victory for abortion rights. Almost 60 percent of voters rejected a referendum to strip abortion rights out of the state constitution, thus enshrining state protections for abortion in the state of Kansas. Voters turned out in record numbers in this deep-red state that Donald Trump won in 2020 by 15 percentage points. Alexis McGill Johnson, president of Planned Parenthood Action Fund, said, "As the first state to vote on abortion rights following the fall of *Roe v. Wade*, Kansas is a model for a path to restoring reproductive rights across the country through direct democracy."

The win was historic and deeply meaningful, but it wasn't a given and it wasn't easy. Activists had formed a bipartisan, broad-based coalition, Kansans for Constitutional Freedom, more than a year before the vote. They raised millions of dollars, outfundraising even the Catholic church's $3 million haul. They pushed for voter registration, helping create a situation in which during the week after *Dobbs* more than 70 percent of newly registered voters in Kansas were women, a trend that held until the referendum. They put up signs and ran ads. They knocked on thousands of doors, made endless phone calls, and held countless living room tea-and-cookie parties, taking the time to explain one on one the deliberately convoluted language of the amendment—a *no* vote meant *yes, keep abortion rights in the constitution.* They had to work to combat misinformation, confusion, conspiracy theories, and outright lies.

A lot of people worked extremely hard for a long time against deliberately dishonest and underhanded tactics to get Kansas voters informed and to the polls.

Kansas was an example of the lengths to which abortion opponents will go to win and of the power that the proabortion majority has to defeat them. This kind of work needs to continue. We've come to a point in time where we can't just say *I'm not political* or *I don't do politics.* Our lives are at stake. We're on the edge of a disaster, but it's not too late. We know community and grassroots political activism works. When we put ourselves to the task of getting people informed and to the polls, the right people are elected to office who then do the right thing. We can enact change because we are in the majority. Think about how President Obama got elected. Think about how community members in deep-red Kansas came together, educated one another, and pulled one another to the polls using a unique and powerful tactic: the truth. Emily Wales from Planned Parenthood explains that in Kansas antiabortion forces "leaned into a lot of theatrics, and in some cases, outright deceiving messages, wholly intended to confuse people. And it undercut trust. All we had to do was be honest with voters."

> We must stop being cynical about politics and get involved because when we deliver a rational, honest message, change happens.

Justice Alito told us that the power now lies with the states and each of their individual electorates. Now, we have to go out state by state, ballot measure by ballot measure, election by election and take control of that power. Red Kansas showed us that no matter the odds, there is hope.

What We're Up Against: Two Kinds of Voter Suppression

Many people avoid politics because of cynicism. They think, *The electoral process is broken. Elections won't affect anything, so why should I vote?* After all, the majority of Americans support abortion, yet as of this writing, abortion is almost completely banned, about to be banned, or greatly restricted in over half the states in the nation. How did this happen if voters have power?

OBVIOUSLY, SOMETHING IS WRONG. BUT CYNICISM ISN'T THE ANSWER. ACTION IS.

Obviously, something is wrong. But cynicism isn't the answer. Action is. The Brennan Center for Justice points out that "the movements to eliminate abortion and restrict the vote are both undergirded by many of the same powerful forces." These forces include those who want to uphold patriarchy, misogyny, heterosexism, and white supremacy.

> When the rights of the majority are being ignored, fighting for abortion includes fighting for fair elections.

Voter suppression has created a situation in which elected officials do not represent the will of their constituents, and we see this in the abortion fight more clearly than in many other issues. It has been a long road to get here, and the longer we ignore the problem, the harder it will be to fix. In fact, many believe that we are close to a tipping point, the point at which tyranny takes over. The stark divide between what voters want and what their politicians do as it concerns abortion just might be our wake-up call and our opportunity to turn things around. It gives us hope.

In 1965, the Voting Rights Act was passed to ensure that state and local governments with a history of discrimination could not pass laws or policies that deny American citizens the equal right to vote based on race. On June 25, 2013, in *Shelby County v. Holder*, the Supreme Court revoked a key provision of this civil rights law. Sherrilyn Ifill, past president of the NAACP Legal Defense Fund, explains that that this created a "wave of voter-suppression laws … around the country with very explicit statements from Republican leaders of those states, saying, 'We're free and clear now.'"

We've seen the results of these efforts, and they're devastating. In 2021, nineteen states enacted thirty-three laws that made it harder for Americans to vote. The Voting Rights Alliance points to sixty-one forms of successful voter suppression, including onerous voter ID laws, closures and reduced access to DMVs so people can't get IDs, failures to accept Native American tribal IDs, failures to accommodate voters with disabilities, elimination of Sunday voting targeted at "souls to the polls" Black voter drives, polling place reductions in marginalized communities leading to hours-long lines, polling place relocations and consolidations leading to confusion, partisan and racial gerrymandering, voter intimidation, and so on.

Researchers at the Brooking Institute point out that "Republican majorities in state legislatures are passing laws making it harder to vote and weakening the ability of election officials to do their jobs. In many states, especially closely contested ones such as Arizona and Georgia, Mr. Trump's supporters are trying to defeat incumbents who upheld the integrity of the election and replace them with the former President's supporters." And things are only poised to get worse. In 2022, there are 245 bills designed to restrict voting that could become law.

In an editorial for *The Washington Post,* Professor Wendy Brown sums up how voting suppression intersects with abortion rights:

> It is also no surprise that while the Court is supposedly turning democracy back to the people in Dobbs, most of the states exalting over this decision are busily de-democratizing themselves by gerrymandering and restricting voting rights in order to restrict minority representation and powers. More than turning a blind eye to these de-democratization strategies, this Supreme Court is actively abetting them. In an earlier decision this season, Merrill v. Milligan, the Court allowed Alabama to use congressional redistricting maps aimed at depowering black voters, maps that a federal court had already deemed illegal, in violation of the Voting Rights Act. The Supreme Court did not bother overturning the federal court decision, just

left it lying in the dirt as it gave the green light to Alabama's redistricting plan.

Despite the odds, we can't give up the fight against voter suppression. Our best tool is to get out and vote now, in every election, for every ballot measure and every amendment, before it's too late. While systemic election reform as of this writing has failed despite Democratic control of the White House, US Senate, and US House—a disastrous result I don't have space to go into here—voting can and does help restore our democracy.

> When deliberate voter suppression succeeds, it leads to another kind of voter suppression—self-suppression.

Those who oppose abortion rights are the minority, and so their goal is to discourage voting. I understand why it works. I see people in my clinic with no government ID, no transportation, no childcare, difficult jobs that don't give time off, and so on. People are wrapped up in their lives, just trying to survive. We need to do better to reenfranchise these people. The National Black Press Association points out that "there are 55 million unregistered Americans eligible to vote, and 10 million are African Americans ... Elections have consequences. The overturned *Roe v. Wade*, the overturned gun laws—are consequences of elections." When we don't come out to vote, we lose. As the National Newspaper Publishers Association president and CEO Dr. Benjamin F. Chavis Jr. put it, "The first form of voter suppression is self-suppression."

This is by design. Voter suppression leads to a sense of hopelessness and cynicism which leads to inaction. It is a deliberate tactic to get people to disengage. I hope knowing that the opposition is making it hard for you to vote on purpose gives you a new sense of purpose. I hope it makes you furious enough to act. The good news is that abortion rights—and voter rights—are now hyperlocal, and that's where grassroots political organizing and voting can work best.

The Importance of Local Politics

What we do at the local level matters because it's the local legislatures that are introducing and passing voter-suppression laws and abortion bans. Here in my home state of Arizona, I've seen this in action. Over 70 percent of Arizonans believe that abortion should remain legal, and yet, as of this writing, we have a slim anti-abortion Republican majority in the state legislature—31 to 29 in the House, 16 to 14 in the Senate. We have just replaced thirteen years of having an antiabortion governor with the election

LAWMAKERS CAN'T BE EXPERTS ON EVERY ISSUE, SO THEY NEED ACTIVISTS AND OTHER MEMBERS OF THE COMMUNITY TO STEP IN TO EDUCATE THEM.

of Katie Hobbs in November 2022. Because of this tiny advantage, the state legislature has been able to introduce copycat bills of draconian abortion restrictions that have found success in other states. For example, they have introduced bills to outlaw medical abortions or to impose "heartbeat" bans. To counter that, we have lobbied against these bills and used grassroots organizing to introduce legislation that's proactive about our reproductive rights. The battle is made more difficult because Arizona is a leader in the sheer number of restrictive voting bills introduced in 2022, making it what the Brennan Center for Justice calls "the epicenter for the fight for voting rights."

It has been a very special experience as an abortion provider to be on the front line of fighting for and against bills while the legislative session is actually happening. As a provider, a nose-to-the-grindstone kind of person, I had been like everyone else, not paying attention until the governor signed something. Then I would talk with my attorneys about how I could come into compliance with whatever new law had been passed so that we could continue to provide abortion care.

Now I'm involved on the front end, and it's been eye opening. Things move very quickly. There's a lot of learning that must happen in a very short period of time, and it has heartened me to find that my medical knowledge and experience as a healthcare provider could make a difference. Lawmakers can't be experts on every issue, so they need activists and other members of the community to step in to educate them.

For example, despite our legislative disadvantage, we were able to help keep the Arizona legislature from banning mifepristone, an abortion drug. We were able to lobby and convince Republican state representatives, one of whom went onto the floor of the state house to support our side based on medical knowledge we helped provide to her. I'm proud that I and other members of our coalition were there to bring this rational, scientific, truthful information to this antiabortion representative that helped convince her that her party's position was too extreme. It wasn't until five months later, on June 25, 2022, that US attorney general Merrick Garland declared that state bans against the drug were illegal, although the legal status of bans is unclear due to not yet being challenged in court. Legislative bans are still being pursued in several states.

Despite beating back several terrible bills during legislative session, one always seems to make it onto the governor's desk. This is how I know that continuously playing defense is the losing proposition. I have a much deeper understanding of how important local elections are, especially in a state like Arizona, where we are so close to gaining control. Our goal is not just to fight antiabortion and voter-suppression legislation but to bring proactive bills to the legislative session to improve access to abortion for Arizonans. One example concerns telemedicine. Because of the pandemic, in December of 2021 the FDA lifted the in-person requirement for medical abortions—the regimen of taking two medications, mifepristone and misoprostol, to end a pregnancy. Yet here in Arizona, we were still requiring people to come to the clinic to have a physician—not even an advanced practice clinician but an actual medical doctor—watch a person take a pill because we had laws previously on the books banning telehealth and requiring that a physician administer mifepristone. In states where providers have access to telehealth visits, people could do the consultations for their medical abortion online, then have their medications mailed to them. Medical abortion has an over 95 percent success rate, and serious complications result in less than one-half of 1 percent of all cases.

I worked with a legislator to introduce a house bill that allowed access to medical abortion care through telehealth appointments without having to undergo an ultrasound unless medically necessary. This was an opportunity for our legislative champions to put forth something that we could all be proud of—a common-sense way to see abortion access expanded in Arizona. However, due to the very small majority of legislators with an extreme agenda, our bill was never even put on the calendar to be debated.

The state legislature is where laws are made, whether about abortion, voter suppression, or other issues that matter.

We have to continue to fight to be in a position where we have the power. In my home state of Arizona, we are so close to being able to take the state house and senate to enact our common-sense, majority-supported bills into law. Robert Draper reports in the *New York Times* that in Arizona, conditions are "the most precarious the G.O.P. has experienced in over a quarter-century as the ruling party. And, of course, Trump lost Arizona in 2020, in large part by alienating the college-educated suburbanites who have relocated to the Phoenix metropolitan area of Maricopa County in increasing numbers … Arizona has thus become what the state's well-regarded pollster Mike Noble characterizes as 'magenta, the lightest state of red.'" In other words, Arizona can once again be a place where people can receive the care they need when they need it, with greater access. And it can be a state where everyone can vote without onerous racist, ableist, and socioeconomically unjust restrictions on who has a voice. We're in there fighting as hard as we can, but we need people to vote in local elections to make our vision reality. Know what's going on in your state and how you can make a difference—before it's too late.

Beyond Voting: Finding Your Lane

After the Supreme Court decision to overturn *Roe v. Wade*, my clinic Twitter feed had several posts from white female abortion providers stating something along the lines of *I'm going to do abortions until they put me in handcuffs and walk me out.* As I've said in these pages before, as a Black woman who is most likely to be the first to be criminalized and the one to suffer the harshest consequences, I'm not willing to go to jail for providing illegal abortion care. Someone called me out for being unsuitably committed to the cause and expressed the sentiment *That's how the Nazis took control.*

We can't all do everything, nor should we be expected to. Everyone must find their own path to how they can best react in light of their own specific conditions, skills, and talents. There are so many ways to show up and support the cause of advancing reproductive health, rights, and justice. There's a place for everyone in this moment. There are many different ways to fight back. If you're willing to go to jail for the cause, or at least to say so on social media, more power to you. For others, our actions may look different. For me, going to jail is not the most effective way to fight back. What I do know is that infighting on social media and calling one another Nazis is definitely not the way to make a difference.

> The majority of people believe in abortion rights, and yet laws are being passed to take away those rights. Getting involved in politics can change that.

Everyone can find their own path to political action, and finding that path starts with getting off social media and getting actively involved in the real world. Stepping outside your comfortable bubble is the first step. My personal evolution from being an academic to becoming an advocate and vehicle for social change was inspired by my deep involvement with the community. My interest in reproductive justice grew as I served and worked with organizations that were working to better the conditions of the community. Once I saw the impact I could have on the conditions of my patients' lives, I knew that my mission was so much bigger than doing a pelvic exam or Pap smear. I saw all the ways in which I could make a broader difference.

In these challenging times, I remind myself that my aspirations for myself when I was young were never just about that one-to-one interaction that a physician has with a patient. It was always about something bigger, always about making a difference in the world beyond that personal connection. The one on one, of course, is very important as a physician, and it keeps me grounded in my understanding of why I do the work that I do. But I always intended to do something greater in the world. To do that, I had to become involved at the level of local, state, and national organizing and policy work. I needed to be sitting at tables with the heavy hitters who have the power to make broad changes to improve the lives of people.

I'm definitely where I want to be at this point in my life, fighting for social and reproductive justice. That mission continues to inspire me to work for social change for Black and Indigenous people and people of color, who are often used as props and talking points about policies but who historically haven't been at the table to affect how these policies are formed. I'm inspired to really get to the root of that, to get knowledge to our communities and give our communities a voice to actively participate in the change that they need to see in their lives. I'm extremely grateful and feel empowered and inspired by every chance that comes my way to make a difference. The more I work, the more opportunities are presented to effect meaningful change. I was invited to appear live on CNN with Jake Tapper to talk about the situation in Arizona and the importance of voting. I was asked what I hope people will do who are upset about our "new normal." I said:

> I really hope that this outrage does translate to more people going to the polls during the midterm election season. What I found since I've been here in Arizona is that a lot of these extreme politicians stay in office in the midterm elections because people don't come out. So the only way that we are going to be able to expand access to care, as opposed to continually having it chipped away at, is we have to have new leadership. We have to have people running our state who are in line with the ideals of nine of ten Arizonans

who believe that abortion should be legal in our state. And so the only way to really turn this around is to vote in champions for the people. In the meantime, we will be doing a great deal of community organizing and mutual aid to mitigate the harms caused by these laws. But ultimately, we need wide policy change at the state level so that we can be protected from votes that happen at the federal level like we've seen with this unprecedented overturn of *Roe v. Wade* at the Supreme Court. And so, we have to demand that the people who represent us and run this state are actually representing our interests.

I will keep repeating that message on as many platforms and in as many places as I can.

To bring the change we want to see, we need to vote and get everyone around us to vote. Vote in every election, no matter how "minor," because right now, it's the small local elections that matter most. Then, educate yourself on the issues that resonate with you and get involved in political action in whatever way works for you. There's a political lane for everyone at this crucial moment in the fight for justice. Disengaging and being cynical about the political process is a luxury we can no longer afford.

> TO BRING THE CHANGE WE WANT TO SEE, WE NEED TO VOTE AND GET EVERYONE AROUND US TO VOTE.

TALKING ABOUT POLITICS:

Myth: People will vote if they care.

Reality: "Kansas showed us that we need money and action to get people to the polls. We can't be complacent because of one win."

Myth: ID laws protect voting integrity.

Reality: "Voter ID laws are presented as ways to fight fraud—but fraud is almost nonexistent. Instead, the real impact of these laws is to disenfranchise people. People with privilege assume that most people drive or have stable addresses. They assume people can get off work to sit for hours in a DMV—if people can even get transportation to their DMV. They assume people have the paperwork they need, like birth certificates or original copies of their social security cards. All that stuff makes voting too hard for people without money or privilege—and that's the point."

Myth: In my blue state, my vote doesn't matter.

Reality: "Katie Porter, Democratic representative for California's Forty-Fifth District, barely won reelection this November. Our votes matter wherever we live."

Myth: In my red state, my vote doesn't matter.

Reality: "When I found out my state was purging voter rolls after missing just a few elections, I realized that staying active is really important. They want to take away our vote, and if we look the other way, they do just that—

legally! They are always planning, so we have to always be voting."

Myth: I'm not a political person.

Reality: "The overturning of *Roe v. Wade* makes clear that everyone's life is political, whether they like it or not. If they can tell me what I can and can't do with my body and my family, there's no separation between me and the state."

Myth: It can't happen here.

Reality: "When Clarence Thomas said that the *Dobbs* decision is a pathway to getting rid of other precedents like gay marriage, we need to believe him. There's nothing stopping the ~~Supreme~~ Extreme Court from doing pretty much whatever they want, so it can happen here. We can't vote out the court, but we can vote out the politicians who actually make the laws."

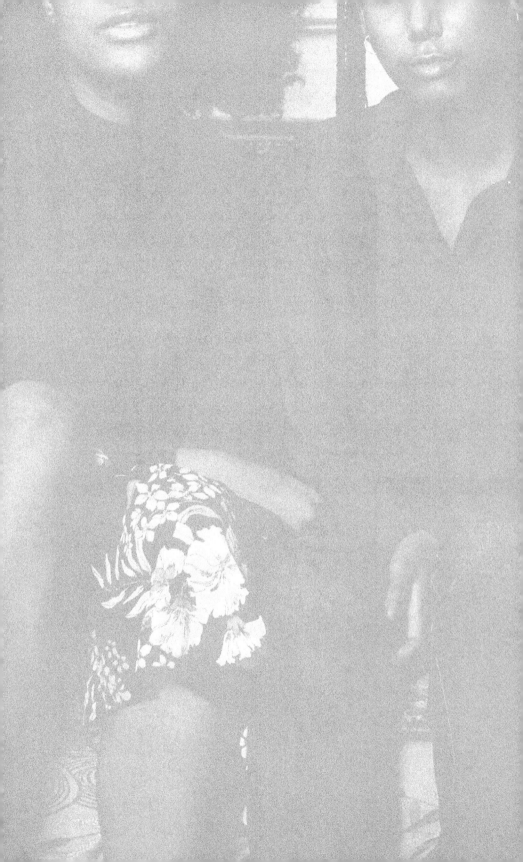

CHAPTER NINE

CREATING AN EMPOWERED FUTURE

About three weeks before I was planning to go to Los Angeles for a personal event, someone I didn't know sent a message to my clinic Instagram account. She and her friends were outraged about what was going on after the defeat of *Roe*, and they were planning an event in Los Angeles to address it. They asked if I could speak or recommend somebody who could. They also wanted me to recommend an organization to raise money for. I don't believe in coincidence. I believe the universe puts things together for us. The stars aligned. Since I was already going to be in Los Angeles that day, I agreed to be their speaker, and we decided to fundraise for my clinic and the Tucson Abortion Support Collective, a group that provides mutual aid for abortion seekers in Arizona.

These three women basically threw a party. The venue was awesome. They had a local DJ and people of all ages and from all different walks of life. There were physicians, other professionals, random friends of friends. It was just a nice eclectic bunch of folks who, for the most part, were pro-choice but had varying understandings of where things stood. I spoke about the situation in Arizona and the rest of the country, where I thought things were going, and what I thought we needed to do about it. The women throwing the event shared information about Plan C, a nonprofit organization that provides information to help people access medical abortion options so they can self-manage their abortion care safely.

People were just blown away by all of it. Many of the guests had thought they knew about what was happening, but by the end of the event, they found out there was so much more to learn and to do. There was something they all could contribute depending on their time, resources, and commitment to the cause. One man came to speak to me toward the end of the party and said, "I just came because I wanted to win the really cool raffle items. And I learned so much."

What these women did that evening is a great example of energized people who had a vision, planned, and made it happen. Plan C, the group they chose to highlight at their party, is a great example of an organization that helps motivated people do just that. Plan C is a "public health meets creative campaign" that envisions a "near future in which the ability to end an early pregnancy is directly in the hands of anyone who needs it." They explain, "Not everyone knows about abortion pills or how they can be accessed online," and so they ask people to "help us spread the word and bring online abortion pill access to the mainstream." They facilitate involvement at every level, from providing stickers that activists can put up around their communities to giving social media guidance to training ambassadors.

If we want to create a better world, we need to envision it, take action, and convince others to join us.

I'm an abortion provider turned reproductive justice activist, so my vision is of a world in which people are empowered to have children, not have children, and to parent the children they have in safe and sustainable communities. This chapter outlines some elements of what that future looks like, what needs to be done to make it happen, and how people can get involved. I focus here on issues that I haven't gone deeply into in previous chapters to show how wide the opportunities for action are, how other movements intersect with the proabortion movement, and how much still needs to be done.

I hope that as you read my vision, you'll form your own vision—as expansive or as focused as inspires you. Then I hope that you'll plan to make that vision a reality. The future truly can belong to us if we put in the work, contribute the resources, and share our visions with others. I saw a glimpse of what that future could look like that evening in Los Angeles. I see it every day when I can serve patients in my clinic with culturally sensitive, justice-inspired care. And I see it taking shape as I join forces with other social justice activists from intersecting movements.

What future do we want to see? What can we do to make it happen? When we all imagine the future that we desire and work together toward that vision, all our stars align, and collectively we make the world the place we want it to be.

WHAT FUTURE DO WE WANT TO SEE? WHAT CAN WE DO TO MAKE IT HAPPEN?

The Vision: A Just Future for Pregnant People

The problem: Pregnant people face barriers to accessing the full range of quality, culturally appropriate care throughout the spectrum of decisions they may make about their pregnancies and birth.

The call to action: Restore, expand, and fund access to abortion care. Expand and fund access to doula services throughout pregnancy and postbirth. Expand state and private insurance coverage for the full range of pregnancy outcomes.

Intersections: Hospitals, physicians, nurses, midwives, doulas, community birth workers, professional organizations, governmental agencies.

My vision of a just future for pregnant people is a world in which they can make informed decisions based on accurate information and then be able to carry out those decisions with accessible and affordable care with the provider of their choice. My role as a physician in creating that vision means bringing abortion care into my general OB-GYN practice, so that it's not siloed into its own arena but is truly just healthcare, like any other service I provide to keep people well. It also means seeing my patients as whole people struggling under various oppressions and helping them access services like Medicaid and having a resource list of organizations that assist with the social systems that can also affect their health, like housing, transportation, and so on. I am called on to be more than a doctor.

My role is also to call out the American healthcare system for its racism and patriarchal structure. History tells us why culturally appropriate care for pregnant people isn't accessible.

Traditionally, birth and abortion care were provided by midwives. The rise of the almost exclusively white male physician in the 1850s when the American Medical Association was established pushed these traditional caregivers out. Criminalization of abortion soon followed to eliminate professional competition, taking women and minorities out of the equation. We need to bring these people back to protect pregnant people from the economically unjust, racist, and patriarchal healthcare situations in which they now find themselves. There is tremendous need for other care providers like full-spectrum midwives, doulas, and community birth workers who can do just this.

To bring them back, we first need to educate the public that these services even exist. Many don't know there is such a thing as a full-spectrum doula who provides both birth and abortion care. Or that there are abortion doulas for people who want just that. These caregivers joyfully step into their historical ancestral roles in assisting people who are pregnant and want to give birth, people who don't want to be pregnant, and even people who can't become pregnant who are going through their infertility journey. This gives me hope for the work we're trying to do to improve maternal and infant health. A post-*Roe* America has shown us that getting back to our roots and our communities works. Community-based practices help people give birth, terminate pregnancies, and raise their children in situations in which they can thrive.

We need to fund these services with private insurance, Medicaid, or other federal and state dollars to expand to meet the needs of our communities. One nationwide poll put the price of doula care between $600 and $2,000 per birth. This expenditure may seem steep for an individual family but actually saves money. People with doula care have fewer cesarean sections and complications. As of 2022, only six states allowed Medicaid to cover doula care with eleven more "working toward it." You probably won't be surprised to hear that states with the strictest abortion bans also typically don't fund or aren't working toward funding doula care. Private insurance is also awakening to the cost savings of providing this service, but again, it's slow-growing and spotty, without mandates or education. We need to teach insurers and the insured that doula services exist and can be beneficial for all.

The Vision: Thriving Communities Where People Can Parent with Dignity

The problem: The fight for reproductive justice includes a person's ability to raise a child in a safe environment, a condition often not met in many communities.

The call to action: Bring together proabortion advocates and groups that promote transportation access and safety, housing security and affordability, environmental protections, pay equity, social safety net expansion and access to services, and so on.

Intersections: Grassroots organizations partnering with corporate, governmental, environmental, and professional organizations.

In a perfect world, we'd see antiabortion forces join us in our vision of thriving communities. Unfortunately, and not surprisingly, this isn't the case. Those of us who support the human right to abortion care are the same people who support affordable housing, a livable wage, access to nutritious food, student debt cancellation, and more. We need to keep our supporters in political power, especially at the local level. So first, as abortion advocates, we need to vote and get involved in politics.

Second, we must bring grassroots community groups together with larger, broader nonprofits and professional organizations. Whatever community you're in, reach outside it. One encouraging thing I've seen since the *Dobbs v. Jackson Women's Health Organization* decision is the larger professional physician and nursing organizations partnering with smaller community advocacy organizations in the name of social justice. Everyone is starting to understand how interconnected all our work is. Instead of everyone going it alone and working in silos, corporate, professional, and other larger groups are reaching into the community, and grassroots groups are welcoming them more and more. Whether you decide to make your voice heard in a larger organization or a grassroots one, reach across the divide to find a partner. We know that change comes from the bottom up. It's the grassroots community that makes it happen. But they also require resources and connections that larger organizations bring to the table. When we work across organizations to help establish frameworks, we can empower advocates on every level.

START WHERE YOU ARE, THEN REACH OUT BEYOND.

Where do you fit into this equation? Start where you are, then reach out beyond.

The Vision: Comprehensive Sex Education

The problem: Politicians use culture-war battles over school curricula for their own personal political gain; extremist forces within communities use sex ed to reinforce historical oppressions.

The call to action: Vote in local and school board elections, pay attention to and get involved in local policy creation, refocus your vision through a reproductive justice lens.

Intersections: Education policy, abortion rights, LGBTQ+ rights, disability rights.

To me, being a doctor was always connected to protecting people. By six or seven years old, I had already decided that I was going to be a physician. In elementary school, I literally became the protector of other girls, the one the kids ran to when they needed help. When I was in the eighth grade, I entered a program for inner city youth who wanted to go into the health field. In high school, there were a lot of pregnant girls. Some had abortions. Others had their babies, and now they're grandmothers. I remember watching all that and thinking that whatever I did with my life, teen pregnancy would be an important part of it. The idea of empowering people who seemed to have no power at all really stuck with me. I had one friend who placed her child for adoption, and in hindsight as an adult, I realized she was wrecked by what happened. These were the kinds of stories that stuck with me.

Still, when I graduated from high school, I had convinced myself that I would be a brain surgeon. It took some time for me to figure out that while brain surgery was a worthy occupation, it was a disconnect from my values, which centered on reproductive rights. By the time I was a sophomore in college, I knew that I would likely be an ob-gyn. Now, I can help people with the sorts of problems I saw derail some of my classmates' lives when I was young. But these problems start long before they come through the doors of my clinic. We need to reach people earlier.

There is no federal requirement that sex ed be taught in schools, so like abortion rights, we face a patchwork of rules and requirements. Beyond some general state guidelines, decisions about sexual education are made by each individual school district. An example of how this often plays out is a regional superintendent in Illinois who said that his parents "are not opposed to offering high school students a 'traditional,' biology-based sex-ed program, but families … don't want all of this other new stuff." By "new stuff," of course, he meant information around LGBTQ+ people; disabled people; gender fluid people; and the racist, homophobic, heteronormative, and other social injustices that underlie the sexual situations kids face. Kids need education that recognizes and honors their intersecting identities, that acknowledges forces of history, and that involves the communities that will be served and impacted. They need sex ed that tells them the truth.

In the United States, 20 percent of thirteen- to fourteen-year-olds and 44 percent of fifteen- to seventeen-year-olds reported that they had "some type of romantic relationship or dating experience." Yet in many states, including Arizona, we currently see state funding that is required to stress abstinence-only sex education, which doesn't work. We need to acknowledge that young people are having sex if we want to help them. There's a concern that if we talk to children about their bodies, they are going to have sex earlier. But when we don't talk to them about their bodies, we're putting them at greater risk for harm.

It's not as scary as our opponents make it out to be. Sex education for preschool and early elementary kids teaches that there are private parts of your body that only you can touch—your body belongs to you. If someone's making a small child feel uncomfortable, now they have trusted adults they can talk to. Kids need to know they have the power to go to their parents to say "I don't like it when Uncle Joe hugs me" or "I don't like to sit on Uncle Joe's lap," so that parents can make the call to stop the interaction. It's not about having sex but about touching, body contact, body autonomy, and personal space.

Preteens need to learn about their changing bodies so that they understand what they're feeling and experiencing. Children assigned female at birth need to be taught about menstruation so that it's not a surprise. Children assigned male at birth need to be taught about erections and wet dreams. All teens need to be taught exactly how pregnancy happens so they can avoid it. I've seen grown women in my clinic who don't really understand anything beyond that they weren't supposed to have sex. They know that at some point, sex ends in pregnancy, but they don't quite know how that happens. I wonder sometimes if a lot of the

WHEN KIDS KNOW WHAT'S GOING ON INSIDE THEM, THEY CAN REDUCE THEIR RISK.

confusion over "life begins at conception" has to do with the lack of understanding of basic biology. When science isn't understood, extreme forces can create their own "facts."

All preteens need to be taught that people other than heterosexuals exist. There's a huge flawed movement created because conservatives believe that teaching about gay, lesbian, bi, and trans people will turn people gay, lesbian, bi, or trans. It's just ridiculous. That's not how bodies work. What we do know is that when kids know what's going on inside them, they can reduce their risk from predators and avoid the mental health issues that arise from feeling there's something wrong with them. Kids faced with confusing feelings often turn to drugs, suicide, and other dangerous behaviors that sex ed can help them avoid.

There's an erasure in sex ed around disabled people that also needs to be addressed. There's an assumption that just because people are wheelchair bound or have different cognitive abilities, they don't have sex or can't be sexually taken advantage of. I will never forget being involved in the care of a pregnant paraplegic woman. I remember thinking, *Well, of course. Just because her arms and legs don't work doesn't mean her reproductive functions are affected.* We need to teach everyone about their bodies and about sex.

We also need to acknowledge racist, sexist, ableist, and heterosexist history so kids can understand what consent looks like. There are a totality of issues that come with having a certain kind of body. When kids are taught that it wasn't until 1993 that the marital rape exception was abolished in all fifty states, about the forced sterilization of populations due to race or disability, or the history of slavery and its ongoing consequences on Black bodies, they can better understand and react to what they see and face in their everyday lives.

Sex ed allows children to understand how to handle the world they live in with knowledge and power.

The reproductive justice framework helps us create sex education that teaches a culture of bodily autonomy that includes all bodies: youth, disabled, LGBTQ+, Black, and so on. It acknowledges that all bodies come with their own history and legacy of how that body has been treated. We're operating from a place where we want all people to thrive. Accurate information and access to resources creates children who grow into responsible members of our greater community.

Because sexual education is decided at the school district level, better sex ed starts with parents. It's ironic that many of the same people who believe a zygote is a fully formed, independent person also believe that kids are their property with no rights of their own to accurate, scientific, fact-based education. The community needs to be involved to set policy to protect kids from this kind of ignorance. It takes everyone, because while many parents are good parents trying to do the right thing, some are not. We see situations all over America where school personnel are mandated to "out" LGBTQ+ kids who confided in them to their parents. We don't need our teachers and counselors forced to be participants in state-mandated oppressions.

Getting involved in local school boards and other local elections is the only way to stop this kind of policy.

The Vision: Decriminalization of Healthcare

The problem: Doctors and other providers are being co-opted into participating in state oppression that targets pregnant people—especially people from marginalized groups—for criminalization.

The call to action: Organizing healthcare workers and allies in refusing to participate in the criminalization of people seeking medical care; harnessing reproductive justice principles to address healthcare issues from a human rights standpoint.

Intersections: Proabortion groups and abolition movements, healthcare workers, hospitals, professional organizations.

> "Who do you serve, who do you protect? Doctors and nurses are not soldiers. Antibiotics are not bombs, hospitals are not the front lines, hard-working medical trainees are not 'gunners,' and neither disease nor patients are 'the enemy.' Militarized language valorizes aggression and violence in medical training and the clinical encounter while obfuscating the loyalties of health workers who serve and protect individuals and communities in need."[80]

Language matters. It affects the way that attitudes, actions, and ultimately, policies, are shaped toward justice or injustice. This narrative in medicine is so pervasive that I even talk about my work "on the front lines." The question of whom we serve and whom we protect demands answering by healthcare workers more urgently now than ever. Not only workers, but who do our hospitals, clinics, universities, and other institutions serve and protect? The more poignant question is whom should we serve and protect?

In an amicus brief presented to the Supreme Court in the *Dobbs* case that overturned *Roe*, concerned attorneys, researchers and others pointed out that "criminalization of reproductive outcomes has devastating, even life-threatening, consequences. It prevents people from

---

80   Iwai et al. https://www.ncbi.nlm.nih.gov/pmc/articles/PMC7365639/#:~:text=Abolition%20
      medicine%20means%20challenging%20race,inaccurate%20notions%20of%20biological%20race

seeking medical care when they need it, subjects them to cruel and humiliating investigations in the midst of medical emergencies, and consigns them to stigma and condemnation in their communities. Worse, the harms of criminalization are disproportionately borne by people who are already marginalized due to racism, sexism, and socio-economic disadvantage."

People often don't realize that every law passed to curtail abortion access creates opportunities to criminalize providers and pregnant people. As the main institutional contact with these people, our job as medical and medical-adjacent providers is to welcome, protect, and help people, not to surveil and potentially criminalize them. We are not extensions of the state. When I became a doctor, I took an oath to do no harm. When I allow myself to be co-opted into the police and carceral state, I am acting against that oath. Members of the health-care community can fight against increased criminalization of healthcare by following the "do no harm" principles set out by decriminalization advocates. From the important work of these advocates, I've identified four main principles for my personal day-to-day clinical work and my personal activism:

> **I TOOK AN OATH TO DO NO HARM. WHEN I ALLOW MYSELF TO BE CO-OPTED INTO THE POLICE AND CARCERAL STATE, I AM ACTING AGAINST THAT OATH.**

1. **Don't call law enforcement on suspicion of fraudulent identification.**

    Our job is to provide healthcare, not to determine whether somebody is undocumented or misrepresenting themselves. Having government-issued identification should have no bearing on people's access to healthcare. Asking healthcare providers to contact law enforcement when they suspect people of trying to fake documentation becomes another reason for people who need care to avoid seeking it, leading to worse outcomes. We know from experience that the people most suspected and turned over to law enforcement will be people from marginalized groups including immigrants, people of color, and trans people whose current identity does not match their birth documents. These, of course, are the very people who often need access to healthcare most. Bringing law enforcement into the healthcare environment is almost never the right choice, and healthcare providers have "no affirmative legal obligation to inquire into or report to federal immigration authorities about a patient's immigration status."

2. End ICE presence in hospitals and in or near healthcare facilities.

Immigration and Custom Enforcement officials have no place in healthcare environments. We know that even lawful immigrants are increasingly fearful of interactions with police and ICE, and thus when they worry about these forces' presence, they avoid seeking care. In order to protect patients from ICE presence, providers should be aware of their rights. This area of law is constantly changing and can be regional, but in general, healthcare clinics are considered "sensitive locations" where ICE activity is limited. Still, providers should be wary of collecting immigration status information and be aware of what documents are in "public view" in case of ICE presence.

3. **Don't support prosecution in cases against people who manage their own care.**

   The majority of people who manage their own abortion care do so successfully. Medical abortion, especially, is extremely safe and effective, and many people are able to perform it with little to no professional intervention. Other ways to self-induce abortions can be less safe and effective, but people still turn to these methods in situations of desperation when no other care is available. When something does go wrong, people need to feel able to go safely to emergency rooms or other providers for help. When we criminalize these people, they won't access care, causing unnecessary injury, illness, or even death. Committing to providing care with no questions asked is crucial in keeping these people safe.

4. **Organize against substandard care in jails, prisons, and detention facilities.**

   Early in my career, I trained at a county hospital where we would have people in labor shackled to beds. I remember asking the guard, "Where's she going to go? She's in labor." Sometimes the guards would unshackle the person. Other times, they refused. I've had patients come from detention for abortion care, and they'd position one guard outside the exam room door and one person inside. I understood that they did this for my safety, but there was no privacy for the person. When a guard wants to be in the room for a surgical abortion, I say, "The person is sedated. What do you think they're going to do?" Pregnant people deserve to serve their time and get the care they need with dignity. Women are the fastest growing population in American prisons, and 80 percent of women in jail are already mothers. Thus, as healthcare providers, we need to really think about what it means when women and mothers go to jail. The ultimate solution is to stop trying to solve social problems with incarceration, and that should be a focus of activism. Until that day, medical providers need to lend our voices to support advocates like Alexa Kolbi-Molinas, deputy director of the ACLU Reproductive Freedom Project, who points out that there is a "lack of universal standards and a range of approaches by authorities governing jails and prisons, as well as the different health care provided ... There is far too little space for accountability, and far too much space for discretion." As healthcare providers, it is our responsibility to fill this space with our voices.

Creating Your Future

We're in a moment right now where just being mad is no longer an option. Everyone needs to define their vision, then find their lane. You can determine your own level of comfort and the options and issues that are in your wheelhouse. There's something you can do right now based on your station in life, ability, intellect, financial resources, geography, and so on. Every person needs to look at the social ills that they're faced with based on their own lived experience and make a commitment to learn more about them, share what they have learned, and find a way to get themselves plugged in so they can work for change. The idea that someone else is going to do it, that the courts are going to take care of it, or that common sense will prevail is over.

My vision of an ideal future is one in which everyone thinks deeply about what they want to see happen and then works toward that goal. I know my life has been greatly enriched by being a part of the solution. I know that yours can be too.

TALKING ABOUT A VISION FOR THE FUTURE

Myth: The opposition's vision stops at getting rid of *Roe*.

Reality: "Pro-life extremists won't stop until a fertilized egg is considered a fully formed person with all the rights that entails. My vision is of a world in which a pregnant person is considered a fully formed person with all the rights that entails. I'm in the majority. I can prevail. But it will take work."

Myth: Comprehensive sex ed encourages people to be gay or trans.

Reality: "I'm only half joking when I say that my vision is to require sex ed for parents so they can learn basic biology about how bodies work. We need to shout scientific facts from the rooftops: sexual orientation and identity is biological, not a matter of personal choice. Kids these days are starting to understand that. The parents, unfortunately, are way behind."

Myth: Teachers, doctors, nurses, and others in positions of power are agents of the state.

Reality: "When I realized that I was being co-opted to enforce historical oppressions, I leaned into my power to resist. Every small decision makes a difference.

Sometimes, it's just protecting one person on one day. But that's how change happens, one small action at a time."

Myth: Proabortion activism only means fighting for choice.

Reality: "Principles of reproductive justice showed me I need to center my efforts on the most vulnerable. To me, that was pregnant people caught up in the prison system. It's brought me unexpected allies and renewed purpose."

CONCLUSION

When I started writing the introduction to this book, *Roe v. Wade* was still the law of the land. By the time I got to this conclusion, *Roe* was gone and the future of abortion in America had entered a new, uncharted territory. In just those four months, I've had to go back to revise these pages over and over to correct for ever-changing circumstances. At each change, I've either rejoiced or mourned. One moment, the successful Kansas amendment enshrining the right to abortion in that state's constitution raised my spirits. The next, I was brought low by the enforcement of an old Arizona statute banning all abortion except to save the life of the pregnant person. I've woken up some mornings not sure I'd be able to keep my clinic operating. And I've gone to bed later that night full of renewed hope from the outpouring of love and support from my community.

WE MUST INTERROGATE OUR OLD WAYS OF THINKING AND REPLACE THEM WITH NEW MODES THAT ARE BETTER SUITED TO TODAY'S CHALLENGES.

One element that has remained constant through all the flux has been that even though we've seen *Roe* fall, the mainstream media and most mainstream advocates are still talking about abortion in the same way they always have. They're fighting the fight with the same tools they tried before. They're again doing all the things that brought us to the place we are now. Times change, and we must change with them when we talk about abortion. In chapter 6, I laid out the new language of reproductive justice and explained why pro-choice is no longer a viable way forward. We must interrogate our old ways of thinking and replace them with new modes that are better suited to today's challenges. If we've learned anything from what's happening now, it must be this.

I'm Pro-Choice, But ____

At a recent talk, I asked the audience to think about how people often qualify their pro-choice mindset by completing the phrase "I'm pro-choice, but ____." The attitudes that arose highlight why we're where we are now and why we need to pivot from the pro-choice debate. As you read these, interrogate your own thinking. How many of these conditions do you put on your support of abortion care?

1. **I'm pro-choice, but people shouldn't use abortion as birth control.**

   Nobody in my decades of experience as an ob-gyn and abortion provider has ever said "Oh, I could get this IUD, but I'll just use abortion instead." That's just not a thing. But even if it was, why are we so concerned about what other people are doing with their bodies? It's none of our business. I could get into all the reasons people don't use birth control. Some can't for medical reasons, others for financial reasons. Most don't because their lives are too complicated, the barriers for access are too steep, or they just don't think they will get pregnant. I could get into the fascinating story of the state of male birth control, which gets stopped in its tracks every time due to the unacceptable side effects, the sort that women and others with uteruses put up with every day from their birth control.

But at the end of the day, other people's birth control is not anyone's business but their own. If we talk about the reasons that people don't use birth control, then we invite strangers and the state into someone else's abortion. We don't want to further the narrative that someone else's abortion is anyone else's business but the person having it. Anything less leads us back to blame, judgment, stigma, and the fact that someone who needs an abortion will not have access.

2. **I'm pro-choice, but why not just have the baby and place it for adoption?**

This statement is really saying "Why not just continue the pregnancy?" The assumption is that the person just doesn't want to become a parent. But there are many people who don't want to be pregnant. In other words, abortion is a pregnancy issue. Adoption is a parenting issue.

Pregnancy can be dangerous for people under the best of circumstances. Childbirth is dangerous. We have the worst maternal mortality rates of so-called developed countries. We do not create the conditions for people to safely make it through pregnancy and childbirth, especially Black people who die at *three to six times* the rate of white Americans, depending on the state they live in. Furthermore, not only can bodies be damaged in pregnancy, but jobs can be lost. Families—especially those with no or insufficient insurance—can be thrown into poverty. The flawed thinking in "just adoption" ignores that someone should be able to choose for themselves whether they want to take those risks with their life, their bodies, and their economic situation. They are not incubators for the use of a potential life.

Because adoption is a parenting issue, not a pregnancy issue, we know that when someone makes it through pregnancy and delivers, they are generally going to parent. People generally don't want to birth a child and then give it away to a random stranger. People glorify adoption. And while many adoptions are wonderful, many are not. Children end up in foster homes and in the child welfare system, with all the problems that entails.

Confusing pregnancy issues with parenting issues is muddled thinking.

3. **I'm pro-choice, but multiple abortions are a sticking point with me.**
Having an abortion is safer than continuing a pregnancy and going through childbirth, so why does it matter that someone has multiple abortions? If one abortion is okay, then more must be okay. We must unpack the thinking behind why this is so hard for some to accept.

Implicit in judging a person for multiple abortions is the judgment that this person is irresponsible. They must be having sex without thought or care about the consequences. You know, sort of like men. Men have been allowed to enjoy sex without shame or consequence for millennia. So, at its core, judging people for multiple abortions is about judging people for their "unacceptable" sex lives.

The idea that women have sex to procreate is a religious value. Why can't women have sex for pleasure without the specter of forced birth? Decoupling sex from pregnancy is only possible when we decouple sex from religious dogma. We need to stand up and say, "Women get to have sex and not be forced into birth if they become pregnant from it." Let's face it, the better the sex, the more of it we have, thus risking the possibility of multiple abortions. People are scandalized by this mode of thinking, but scandal only arises when judgment is involved. We need to stop judging and let people be. A friend of mine likes to say, "Every sperm does not have to have a name." Neither does every fertilized egg.

4. **I'm pro-choice, but I wouldn't have an abortion myself.**
   This statement is rarely true. Often in my clinic, I see people who say they never thought that they would be here making this decision. I tell them that abortion is very common. I ask, "Why do you believe so strongly that you would not have an abortion when one in four people who can become pregnant will have an abortion?" What makes these people think they're any different? When we set ourselves apart, we "other" the folks who do have abortions, when really, they're just like us, not somehow inferior or less moral. They are very likely making a good and moral decision for themselves and

for their families, just like you might if you were ever faced with the prospect of an unintended or unwanted pregnancy. They are everyday people making everyday decisions in the midst of complicated lives, just like you or someone you love could be. No one knows for sure what they'll do until they actually confront an unwanted pregnancy. When it comes down to their own well-being, people will do what is right for their specific situation. I hope this gives people pause before they judge others and set themselves apart.

5. **I'm pro-choice, but within reason.**

These are the people who are okay with abortion restrictions. For example, maybe they're comfortable with an abortion ban beyond fifteen weeks except in the case of rape, incest, or danger to the life of the pregnant person. That sounds "reasonable." But then, what do you think will happen to that ten-year-old who's twenty-three weeks pregnant by her father? Who's going to do that abortion? Who will do the abortion of that twenty-week pregnant woman who just found out that her fetus has heart, lung, brain, kidney, and genetic defects that are incompatible with life and the delivery might put her own life in danger?

In reality, most healthcare professionals aren't willing to risk their licenses or to go to jail because of the complicated nature of what "life of the mother" means. We've seen this already with professionals refusing to perform abortions until a truly dire emergency exists—sometimes too late. We see providers moving out of states where "life of mother" exceptions exist, thus putting care out of reach of people who will need emergency care. We see clinics in states with these bans closing in record numbers, further limiting access to care.

Even the doctors who stay may not be much help. There has to be the opportunity to gain the skill set and expertise to safely perform those unique, special abortions that you think are okay. Healthcare professionals won't have the skills to perform abortions later in pregnancy if they're so severely restricted. They won't be able to train the next generation of doctors. It takes training and experience to take care of those very particular, specific cases. The way healthcare providers learn to treat people is to actually have people to treat.

You can't have it both ways. As soon as there is any restriction, it becomes too risky for the practitioner and for the emergency patients they're expecting to be helped, and soon, the skills are atrophied. Allowing for "reasonable" restrictions means when people need help, it won't be there. Any restriction is a recipe for unnecessary harm.

Healthcare and Criminalization

As we see from "I'm pro-choice, but _____" attitudes, seeing abortion through a pro-choice lens has allowed us to "other" people who we think are not like us and to compartmentalize special cases and specific people, as if we're not all in this together when, really, we are. When we abandon the pro-choice lens and look through the reproductive justice lens instead, we stop seeing individuals and their individual circumstances and start seeing communities and the intersections between abortion rights and the wider fight for human rights. We realize that we're all in it together.

Nowhere is this more dire than in the issue of criminalization of abortion care. As soon as there is any restriction on abortion, there are mechanisms for the state to enforce those restrictions. That brings the state and the carceral system into the exam room and into our personal lives. When we criminalize medical professionals and people who become pregnant—and now in some cases even their friends and family who aid them in seeking care—there can be no middle ground.

REPRODUCTIVE JUSTICE CAN MOVE US FORWARD.

Be proabortion. "I'm pro-choice, but ____" brought us here, in part. Reproductive justice can move us forward.

Abortion Care Is Healthcare

Abortion care is healthcare, even when not all healthcare professionals want to provide it. Honestly, I'm not interested in removing gallbladders. What I ask from other healthcare professionals is to support a pregnant person's decisions about how they want to care for their own body. Also understand that even if a doctor wants to provide abortion care, we still must staff our clinic to provide the care. Each person from the receptionist to the medical assistant to the person who has the specialized training to start an IV or administer medications to the janitor who cleans up at night are subject to the stigma and harassment that has been mainstreamed regarding abortion.

"I'm pro-choice, but____" thinking allows the media and the general public to focus on rare, "tragic" cases, because these are what get clicks and what arouses emotional responses, making for good fundraising and self-righteous indignation. However, these are not the stories we should be calling attention to. Sure, as a practicing ob-gyn, I've seen my share of people in dire situations. But more often, this isn't what I hear and understand about the struggles pregnant people face. What I see is not usually the story the media tells of a tragedy that can be solved with a quick cross-state trip. It's not even the story that will be solved by making abortion legal in most cases. Instead, I hear the kind of everyday strain of people who want to stay in school. Or people who can't care for more children because they're already just scraping by caring for the children they already have. Or people who are just too young to have a child of their own.

> Abortion is common. It's every day. One in four people capable of giving birth will choose to have an abortion at some point in their life.

These people come to me on any typical Tuesday afternoon without any headlines or tragedy. They know what I know: that abortion care is safe and low risk. They don't even really need a physician for a medical abortion, honestly, even though they're often glad that I'm there with them to answer their questions and listen to their stories. Most people who arrive at my clinic to get abortions aren't distraught when they show up. Most people who leave my clinic aren't weeping. They're relieved and heading right back to their jobs, their partners, and their children.

The exceptions and tragic cases are absolutely heart wrenching, but our focus on those erases ordinary people who have abortions for ordinary reasons. It erases the fact that people generally have abortions because it's just not the right time to add to their family or to start a family. This is the everyday story. The one nobody wants to tell because it doesn't get clicks online. It doesn't drive people to the voting booth, or make people take out their checkbook in a fit of pro- or antiabortion fervor.

My message, and the message that reproductive justice delivers, is this: Abortion care is healthcare. It's routine and it's common and has been for millennia and will continue to be moving forward, no matter the law. Abortion care is healthcare because denying access to abortion makes people, families, and communities sicker, both physically and mentally. Abortion care is healthcare if a pregnant person is facing death, if he wants to finish his bachelor's degree, or if she wants to be able to afford to feed the children she already has. Abortion care is healthcare, whether the fetus has a genetic abnormality or if the pregnant person knows that their partner is about to leave them. Abortion care is healthcare, always, because as soon as we talk about it as anything less than the basic human right to the care of our own bodies, families, and communities, there will always be a politician or activist judge wanting to step in and make laws in their best interest, not in ours. If abortion care isn't healthcare, then these people will always be the ones who will get to decide who "deserves" an abortion and who doesn't.

We need to stop talking about regulating abortion and being "pro-choice, but _____" and instead talk about how we can ensure all people have the right to not have children, to have children, and to parent any children they have in safe and healthy communities.

In other words, we need to be talking about reproductive justice, a conversation that centers the everyday situations of everyday people struggling with forces outside their control: unaffordable day care, lack of access to healthcare, insufficient paid time off, unsafe communities to raise children, a nonliving wage, and so on.

Abortion care needs to be available for everyone in all circumstances.

"I'm pro-choice, but _____" rhetoric allows for "good" versus "bad" abortions, thus creating stigma and shame. Every abortion someone decides to have is valid when we respect the humanity of the person who is pregnant. Do you really value the embryo and fetus over the life of the person that is required to eventually birth it? What is really stopping you from being proabortion? Anything less takes us back to where we failed before.

Anything less leaves someone, their family, and their community sicker, poorer, and devoid of hope. No abortion ban is acceptable. *Abortion care is healthcare. Abortion care is healthcare. Abortion care is healthcare.* That is the message I, as a physician who provides abortions and as a reproductive justice advocate, am determined to deliver to the world.

You already know and love someone who has had an abortion. If you don't think you do, then I hope that what you have learned in the chapters of this book helps you become someone who can be trusted with the abortion stories of the people you love. Give yourself the permission to be unabashedly proabortion.

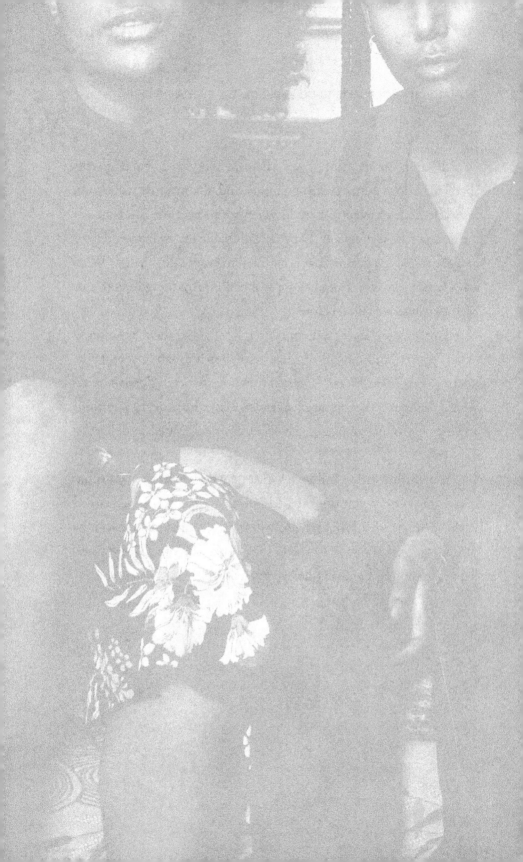

ABOUT THE AUTHOR

Dr. DeShawn Taylor, MD, is an award-winning gynecologist and family planning specialist, gender-affirming care provider, associate clinical professor, and reproductive justice advocate whose work advances reproductive healthcare access through direct services, education and training, advocacy, and leadership. She envisions a world where people can access the full range of just, culturally appropriate, and exceptional reproductive healthcare regardless of their circumstances or zip code.

As founder and CEO of Health Justice MD, Dr. Taylor helps organizations incorporate a justice lens into new and emerging commitments to support reproductive rights. Recognized by the Maricopa County NAACP as a trailblazer and as a champion of choice by the National Institute for Reproductive Health, Dr. Taylor sees patients at her Desert Star Family Planning clinic and facilitates coalition work with her nonprofit, Desert Star Institute for Family Planning, in Phoenix, Arizona. The Religious Coalition for Reproductive Choice awarded Dr. Taylor and her clinical staff the Dignity to Decide Award that honors prophetic action and leadership that challenges the status quo in service of reproductive freedom and dignity.

Born, raised, and trained in Los Angeles, California, Dr. Taylor received her MD degree from UCLA, OB/GYN training at King/Drew Medical Center, and complex family planning training with an MS degree in clinical and biomedical investigations—patient-oriented translational research at USC. In her free time, Dr. Taylor prioritizes rest! She enjoys listening to audiobooks and morning jogs to start the day when the Arizona weather is mild.

GET IN TOUCH

You may contact Dr. DeShawn Taylor by visiting the websites of her various organizations. If you need clinical care or would like to support the activities of the Desert Star Family Planning clinic, please visit www.desertstarfp.com. For inquiries regarding tax deductible donations or information regarding the programs provided by the nonprofit Desert Star Institute for Family Planning, visit www. desertstarfp.org. Organizations looking to engage with Dr. Taylor for consulting services should visit www.healthjusticemd.net, where you can also read blog posts inspired by this book.

CPSIA information can be obtained
at www.ICGtesting.com
Printed in the USA
JSHW052050100723
44489JS00001B/1

9 781642 256598